Living Consciously: The Science of Self

Kingdom of God
Virtue
Yellow
Immortal
Communism
Folly
Enemy
Catholic
Vice
Animal
Child
Death
Not Me
Daughter
Mother
White
Philosophy
Weakness
Strength
Air
Criminal
Management
Labor
Education
Insanity
Jew
Brother
Wife
Space
Fire
Anarchy
Psychology
Capital
Between-ness
You
Bad
Infidel
Son
Democracy
God
Hell
Man
Heaven
Mineral
Body
Self-Consciousness
Moon
Ignorance
Motion
Sex
U.N.
Judge
Origin of Life
Atheist
Electron
Husband
Good
World
Protestant
Water
Father
Sister
Religion
Black
Woman
Blood
Time
Vegetable
U.S.A.
Star
Imagination
Devil
Atom
Life

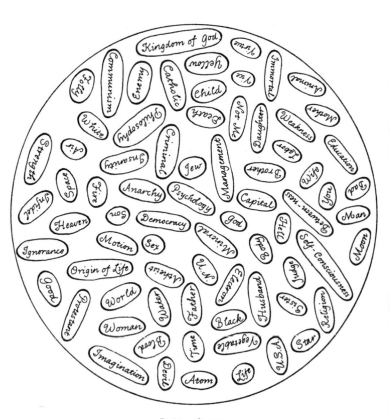

I, Myself, Me

John M. Dorsey and Walter H. Seegers

LIVING CONSCIOUSLY:
THE SCIENCE OF SELF

Detroit—Wayne State University Press—1959

Second Printing, December 1965

To My Humanity

PREFACE

THIS book has been written as a demonstration of the fact that scientific data can be claimed and recorded as self-data, as actual creations of the scientist. Its purpose is to attest the health benefit inherent in considering scientific education research and service as the self-activities of a given scientist.

For more than a decade, we have worked closely together in the field of health education, our medical school departments (physiology and psychiatry) being particularly responsible for providing the scientific facts of normal human development. The following truths gradually became clearer and clearer (and correspondingly life strengthening) to both of us:

Wholesome education is the student's conscious effort to use his mind for developing its usefulness.

The painfully limited hygienic success of formal education to date is traceable to ignorance of and disregard for the reality that everyone's health and happiness depend directly upon the degree to which he achieves the harmonious development of appreciation of his own life's augmenting treasures.

What is now regarded popularly as learning is the only obstacle to the apprehension of the supreme truth that conventional education which does not systematically fea-

ture knowledge as self-knowledge does systematically en-
force health deviation (illness).

The impersonal appearance of conventional language
is blindly trusted and firmly established. It is so misleading
that one who uses traditional word forms cannot behold
himself while utilizing his own self-activities. To attain
and maintain self-awareness each of us authors has had to
develop and practice a vocabulary clearly respecting the
comprehensiveness of his enlarging individuality. We had
to do this as an indispensable stepping stone to assuming
the right use of our minds. But for ease in reading, our
language generally conforms to standard usage, even
though a certain semantic psychosis is involved.

We daringly decided to risk the reading public's dis-
approval by painstakingly writing this book unconvention-
ally in the first person singular. Actually, this is the only
case and number which realistically uphold the allness of
oneness, the entirety of individuality. We have even tried
to devise a signature form indicating authorship which
observes the sameness, or equality, of personal identity.
Each author lives all that he designates as "his own fellow
author" and considers himself sole author of all of his
living (including this work).

To spare ourselves superfluous pain, our many-times-over
tested and validated scientific findings are, and must be,
presented specifically as having proven helpful to ourselves
alone—and as having no other possible claim upon our
reader. By concentrating upon the single fact of his own
life, each of us gradually succeeded in healthfully extending his appreciation of his own life.

From the works of men who have studied human individuality, notably those of Freud, we have evolved for ourselves the following hypothesis which we have been subjecting to every conceivable test for its *particular* applicability: Everyone is grievously ill on account of his limited self-appreciation and can become well only by extending the scope of his self-tolerance with self-love. This hypothesis passes *every* test. It works. It does not work only where it is not tried. Its practicality and utility for everyday living is demonstrable in every instance of its application. It is offered as the chief desideratum of a world constantly troubled by hot, or cold, warfare. In the opposite direction, efforts at self-ignoration would reverse the life order and are helpfully signalized by inharmonious living, which leads to the misprision of life itself. In view of its being a common addiction, self-disesteem is rated as natural or healthy, but as anyone grows a fuller view of his wonderful creative power his life's all-precious worth becomes constantly self-evident.

We have not been able to discover any flaw in our scientific orientation that "all observation is self-observation." On the contrary, we have felt keenly the wonder that we so long resisted a vital truth so obviously simple and salutary. The consideration of prevailing educational methods reduced our wonder to guilt; and self-love reduced our guilt to responsibility.

We have helped ourselves thoroughly by reading and make extensive use of quotations. Numerous authors and publishers, present and past, have thus been most helpful. We wish to acknowledge, particularly, the permission of *Harper's Magazine* for the quotations from P. W. Bridgeman's essay which appeared in the March, 1929 issue; the permission of the Philosophical Library for the quotation from Max Planck's *Scientific Autobiography and Other Papers;* the permission of Methuen and Company, Ltd., for the quotation from Alexander Moszkowski's *Einstein The Searcher;* and the permission of E. P. Dutton and Co. for the quotation from *Freedom and Growth and Other Essays* by Edmond Holmes.

John M. Dorsey
Walter H. Seegers

CONTENTS

PROLOG

EVER SINCE Freud's vital discovery of his valid and epoch-making method which enables a human mind to strengthen and heal itself by means of the extension of its power of consciousness, every kind of antagonism regarding it has appeared. Such antagonism toward life-consciousness, technically recognized as resistance which is always traceable to self-intolerance, has been found to be a regular forerunner of conscious life-affirmation. An untrained mind is not capable of immediate intuitive appreciation that its own modifications account for all of its living of its mental powers. As a corrective, the systematic study and practice of conscious individual living develops mental insight which is the essence of mental health.

The systematic practice of self-insight is required to free a person from viewing himself as a tool, a means, developed for the sake of something outside of himself. Devotion to the work of extending his consciousness of his own life is necessary to affirm a person's realization of his life as being an end unto himself. Than this perfection of self-appreciation there can be no greater, except the all-meaningful success of being alive itself.

Self-activity, then, is the life-saving truth hidden in the illusion of acquiring knowledge, instead of creating it. Said Bacon, "Man's nature runs either to herbs or to weeds;

therefore let him seasonally water the one and destroy the other." Changing one's mind (extending its recognized boundaries) in order to tolerate further self-insight is irksome and involves hard work. Only a hard life can develop a strong mind. The preparation of this book has been a most arduous and most rewarding discipline. Every reader originates what he reads. To the extent that he acknowledges this fact and, thereby, extends his life-consciousness, he cannot but reward himself fully for his sufferance. So be it.

My world common man is now imbued with the spirit of science. He conceives this spirit emphatically as having its focus on external facts. His attention to human life activity, as such, is given a subsidiary rank. This kind of science perspective is a sure source of mental trouble, which I can call an attempt at dehumanization. It misplaces the meaning of human sense experience, quite as Max Planck has observed: "Every individual has his own senses, and, in general, the senses of one individual are quite different from those of another, whereas the aim of exact science is to achieve objective, universally valid knowledge. It may seem, therefore, in adopting our present view we have been following the wrong track." I have deluded myself habitually with leaning on "objective, universally valid knowledge," and I feel this comforting habit of mind threatened when I am called upon to consider my reliance upon my *illusions* of externality as the "wrong track." Quite naturally I can resist and be hostile about considering the science of self as the scientific "right track."

The exercise of self-consciousness as a method for evolving the science of self can only be described with the use of

Prolog

a language required for that purpose. This is not easily found, nor am I as author, able to master easily some of the hard facts which I have considered. During a period of more than seven years I wrote this work again and again and know very well that I had to apply myself with great energy. Even more, I am convinced that the health benefits of this science of self accrue to me only when I practice self-conscious activity and devote myself to it steadily. I find that this investment pays great returns—and I had to find that out for myself, too. As Max Planck noticed, "A new scientific truth does not triumph by convincing its opponents and making them see the light."

I have a great need to humanize my science, for I feel the truth of T. North Whitehead's observation, *"I have never met a scientist who had become cultivated (in the humanistic sense) by virtue of his scientific education or by his subsequent work as a scientist."* The science of self is specifically human and the exercise of self-consciousness is its one source.

I. INTRODUCING MYSELF

Self-reverence, self-knowledge, self-control,
These three alone lead life to sovereign power.

TENNYSON

EVEN UPON his first living of the title of this book, my reader may word, as follows, his resistance to working his way to a larger concept of his life through the exercise of his consciousness: "I am sensitive to such words as 'self' or 'selfishness' or 'self-consciousness.' Whenever I suffer an attack of self-consciousness, I wait until it passes over, so that I can go on living myself with my customary self-unconsciousness."

Yet, there is nothing that can be interesting or intriguing but myself. The "I" is the thrilling subject. My hopes, my wishes, my fears, my whole earth, my sky, my sun revolve for me, all are made by and for me. I give birth to myself, I live, and I end my life. How? Why? What? I go to school, go to college, take on (live) my world. How? What for? I buy clothes, I sell clothes, I eat this, I eat that, I walk, I ride, I work, I play, I go east, I go west, I write, I read, I listen, I talk, I love, I hate, I am well, I am sick, I think, I dream, I sleep, I awaken, I never get enough of myself.

So many times I annoy myself with the feeling something is lacking, something is missing. Can it be my restricted self-appreciation?

However, I may seem to know little about myself. I may go through life hardly on speaking terms with myself. Oh, I recognize a photograph of my face but often fail to recognize a photograph of my feet. I know myself by name; but how much do I know the real motives with which I drive myself, the roots of my own likes and dislikes, of my own strengths and weaknesses? Is my apparent lack of self-knowledge due to mental blocking? Why do I deny, evade, and run from certain aspects of me? What is terrible about being conscious of what I am? What is wrong in my acknowledging that all of my knowledge must be self-knowledge?

I may well ask myself, "Have you ever considered sufficiently the full meaning of your individuality? Has the truth of the *allness* of your individuality been lived by you as fleeting thought, undoubtedly occurring at irregular intervals? Has the scientific fact of the inviolability of your personal individuality been the leading health principle of your life, which it wholesomely can be? Why not begin to suspect yourself of self-deception in your ever flagrant habit of living your obviously rejected experiences as if they were outside of you?"

I cherish the story of the child given the task of solving a jig-saw puzzle of his earth. Asked to account for the swiftness of his solution he replied, better than he knew, "Oh, on the opposite side of the blocks there was a figure of a man. When I got my man together right I had my earth right."

Introducing Myself

In observing that I, and only I, make all of my life, I must see that I, and only I, have the power to make myself happy or unhappy, loving and lovable or unloving and unlovable, amiable or angry, and so on. In recognizing my creative power as all mine, I find my scientific imagination in its mental disposition which is most favorable to creative effort.

Conscious self-knowledge (and the seeking of further conscious self-knowledge) is my mind's sovereign remedy. Sovereignty of mind necessitates the development of the ability to reign well.

Every word my reader lives is an activation of his own self-power. Seeing selfness is humanizing selfness; evaluating selfness is deifying selfness. This idea is ever new, yet it is one of the oldest and most repressed ideas in my history of man. Healthful education stems only from this principle of reality.

As a student, my most helpful insight is: man is absolutely unteachable. My description of my learning process, given in this volume, is the fruit of this insight.

This volume aims to establish the health significance of the development of the love of self-tolerance. The extension of self-tolerance is essential for the love of life itself. I can have only one problem of life: How to develop in order to tolerate myself kindly, how to grow to endure my life's ordeals (ultimately) with loving and appreciative endurance. Awareness of my need for tolerance is the product of my sensing my enlarging (growing) identity.

Humanization is the peace cry. Any and every expression of my life admits of being humanized through one process only, namely, through the vivifying process herein described as my consciously living it. Illusions of non-human externality fill in every mental hole created by self-unconscious living.

In what sense then do I use the word "self"? In the sense in which it means *all of only one,* for this is the meaning which I ascribe to every element of life: the whole of it and nothing but it. My self means my unity and my totality. I *must* take my life lightly, figure that I do not amount to much, and generally discount the precious value of my wonderful human being, exactly to the extent that I cannot employ my uniquely human power of self-consciousness.

In this book, therefore, I take the position that I, an individual, include my all. I take the view that my life is all and only about me. *That* is the platform of self-consciousness. Through research I have tried to see the consequences of looking at my life in this manner, and I find that it is to my health benefit to align myself with this natural condition of my creation.

II. ONLY I CAN HELP MYSELF

I am my brother, and my brother is me. If I feel over-shadowed and outdone by great neighbors, I can yet love; I can still receive; and he that loveth maketh his own the grandeur he loves. Thereby I make the discovery that my brother is my guardian, acting for me with the friendliest designs, and the estate I so admired and envied is my own. It is the nature of the soul to appropriate all things. Jesus and Shakespeare are fragments of the soul, and by love I conquer and incorporate them in my own conscious domain. His virtue—is not that mine? His wit—if it cannot be made mine, it is not wit.

EMERSON

THE TERM "science" derives from the Latin word *scire,* meaning to know. By "science" I mean organized (systematic) self-knowledge. Science, as an educational movement, developed out of the need for knowledge free of superstition. *One,* only *one* anything, *can* have a mind, or soul, or self, or consciousness, or life or being,—even two cannot, or three or more. Scientific letter and spirit turn directly on the *literal* and *spiritual* meaning of that organic necessity; human individuality. Health benefit de-

9

rives from my systematically noticing my self-living as being my all. With this accurate self-perspective I can elevate
my self-estimate to a new unity, with every new life experience.

This work sets forth a consistent scheme for making
practical mental conceptions. For instance, the question
of whether or not an external reality underlies mental
phenomena and corresponds with perceptions is not at
all safely and sanely disposable as being merely an academic
question, or an impractical philosophical matter, or a
non-essential metaphysical concern. Quite the contrary;
recognition of the true nature of the specific reality sub-
stantiating natural science discoveries, turns out to be
of the most practical significance for my mind's healthy development. My every scientific method is essentially a way
of discovering order and unification in, not out of, my
human nature. "Thus there is dawning a new view that the
whole of life and the whole ascent of life are interpene-
trated with 'mind.' "—J. ARTHUR THOMSON.

Each scientific method starts with one observed fact after
another, usually ending in a generalization from a limited
number (a fair sample). A chief and deplorable source of
trouble with the use of science as a tool is that, as the
Encyclopedia Brittanica article "Science" records, "science
is not as a rule concerned with individuals as such but with
kinds or classes." It is the enormity of this specific desideratum of my formal science (mind saving recognition
of the universality of individuality) which confirms the
worth of the subject matter of this book. As the stockpile
of self-consciousness increases the stockpile of atomic bombs
decreases.

Only I Can Help Myself

The question arises, Why should I concern myself whether or not a scientist realizes, or is capable of realizing, that his every scientific observation is a self-observation? Why need I bother about the fact that my fellow man on the assembly line does not recognize that management, or his automobile, or his factory, is too in each instance his own living of it? Do I not get the same fine automobile as a product whether or not its worker lived self-consciously? The explanation is sun-clear. Not so many years ago every American citizen deplored the product of slave labor, often boycotting it. But that kind of slavery did not necessarily make a slave. The true slave is the man who is not conscious that he is the author of all of his living, that he is the creator of his all.

I am a pseudo-scientist when I am a slave of my data, when I claim that my data are not my very own life's creations. I am a pseudo-scientist when I live any kind of self-detraction. I am a pseudo-scientist when I do not live every aspect of my scientific living as a means of sensing more profoundly and extensively the self-esteem proper to my human being. I am a pseudo-scientist when I do not consider my ideas and feelings of adoration, reverence, holiness, and divinity as scientifically worthy. Indeed scientific living may be identified with religious living in the all-important sense that each describes the greatest possible human appreciation of being alive. My qualifications of "exact," or "pure," science are, first of all, that it be recognizable as the best means for growing self-knowledge; then, that it be appreciated as my own choice of mental discipline; and finally, that it be lived as my happiest means for realizing and fulfilling the potential of my free, and ever frcsh, life. I seek scientific progress not only on account of achieving the benefits of my disciplined mind, but also on account of avoiding painful signs and symptoms (cries for help) of my untutored mind. That epoch making student of his mind's consciousness, my Sigmund Freud, observed, "I have always thought that self-reliance and natural self-confidence are the indispensable conditions of that which appears to us to be greatness if it has led to success. I also think that a distinction must be made between greatness of achievement and greatness of personality."

The clearest explanation offered by my pseudo-scientist, accounting for his qualifying his definition of science by depersonalizing adjectives (such as "objective," "disinterested," "dispassionate," "impersonal," "physically measurable") is that such qualifications serve as reminders to the scientist to consult his sensory, as opposed to his phantasied, experience. However, such an explanation, by positing an advantage in the undispelled illusion that scientific living is not entirely the scientist's own living, is defensible only at the high cost of promoting unrecognized mental dissociation. The truth is that my scientist lives his sensations, his perception, and his phantasy,—each to the same full extent. Every way in which my scientist lives himself has the same rank insofar as it is all and only his own personal living of it.

Before I can well continue my science of self I need to have a clear view of the meaning of "self," and of "consciousness." By "self" I mean nothing but singleness of human being, nothing but oneness of human individuality. Meaning, itself, can be nothing but a mental construct standing for life value. In other words, the term "self" means all inclusiveness and inviolability of the integrity of human existence in its one and only occurrence in one human existent. For the practical purpose of this work, the term "self" and the term "mind" may be considered synonyms. The term "self," thus considered, provides the definition of the whereabouts in which all living of any meaning (life value) takes place. Thus, I live each and every meaning of my life in my own mind, in my mental living. To grow the self-tolerance to appreciate as I that which before I had to repudiate as not-I, that is mind strengthening. It is not a benefit to maintain two inharmonious parts of my own mind, one of which I nominate "I," the other of which I nominate "not-I." Therefore I use the terms "I," "self," and "mind" as synonyms.

The question which I now may consider is, What difference does it make whether or not I appreciate the truth of my own allness? This question introduces the fact of consciousness, the health importance of consciousness and unconsciousness.

Consciousness is a living of wakefulness, awareness— ultimately of appreciation of being alive. And what am I conscious of? I am and can be conscious only of myself. I cannot be conscious of some other person, chair, star, car, or the hate and love of some other person. Every kind of other is nothing but my own living of it. That is all a part of me. This view exercises my consciousness of myself. Even when I pretend that my otherness is not I, such is only a self-deception. This pretense has, however, been cultivated so extensively, that its exposure in my book is bound to arouse resistance. That resistance alone will make my book difficult to read for the first time. However, I face this resistance and kindly develop a picture of the health values of devoting my attention to the true picture of myself as being my *all there is.*

Seeing my selfness as being my all and only living confronts me with the fact that my consciousness also consists of selfness. My consciousness, though, is all and only about consciousness, and therefore cannot actually be lived as consciousness of anything else. My consciousness (made up of my own selfness) can be lived by me while I am living other parts of myself also. For instance, living my hand or my car at the same time that I live my consciousness, enables me to identify my hand or my car as my own living of it. Furthermore, I am unable to discover any other way for attaining the wholesomeness of self-conscious living.

The true awareness of myself, including my tendency to deceive myself, constitutes my healthful living. How to operate myself—all of me, including what I might dislike or claim is not-I—constitutes the science of self. In the science of self I recognize all there is as being I and proceed to cultivate myself scientifically. I cultivate myself to grow all of myself well. I recognize that it is entirely up to me to see to it that this is done for my greatest happiness. I must work to acknowledge my comprehensive nature and devote myself to proper self-regard. In the science of self I recognize that I am responsible to myself for what I do with myself. In the science of self I increase my exercises of earnestness, seriousness, deep sincerity, careful concern; and I renounce exercises of such feelings as flippancy, recklessness, indolence, suspicion, gloom, stage fright, and envy. In the science of self every day is judgment day. Each one of my (self) unkindnesses is costly but I pay fully for it as I go. Each one of my investments is beneficial and I get what I pay for. Let me ask again, what do I —— consist of; and may my reader insert his own name in the blank space.

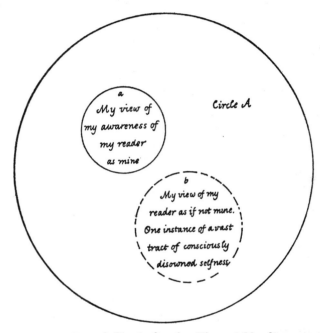

a

My view of
my awareness of
my reader
as mine

Circle A

b

My view of my
reader as if not mine.
One instance of a vast
tract of consciously
disowned selfness

CHART I. *A Comprehensive View of Myself*

My comprehensive view of myself reveals me as *all inclusive,* as being all of my own authority and responsibility. It can accurately be represented as circle A of Chart I. This circle includes all of me—that of which I am aware and that of which I am unaware. My view of my awareness of myself is only a part of my total self and is represented by circle *a* within A. Any new growth creates a new circle *a*. Circle *a* is perfectly integrated with A.

When I live my idea that there is something that is not-I, that very idea is an individuation of my individuality. I create my illusion that there is something that is not-I, and that very illusion is an element of my being. My creation of my illusion of my otherness living is pictured by my circle *b*. In this way I symbolize my living of myself which has been discovered and repudiated. I live my repudiated self as if it were not I after all. Consequently, I live symbol *b* as if it could exist outside of A. Since it is in reality impossible to go outside of myself, to live something that is not I, circle *b* is drawn within circle A. Circle *b* is my outlawed self which is not appreciated as being entirely mine; hence I must notice *b* with discomfort. If my signal of self-disharmony, like my pain of my finger on my hot plate, is not dealt with expertly, more extensive signaling of self-injury is the consequence.

When I regard my reader accurately as an element of myself, as my own creation, I have my view of my awareness of myself—circle *a*. When I regard my reader inaccurately as somebody besides myself, not my own creation, I create my illusion of separation and my illusion of joining—circle *b*. Each illusion is conveniently used. Thus I like to remark about my own trouble as being my reader's. Thus, I would use "crazy" talk and say: "Joe Doe over there is a bad one. He is envious of me and does not want me to succeed." Or, "John Doe over there is a good one. I wish I had some of his success." Or, "Jane Doe is certainly a fine woman; however, a woman must ever be foreign to me since I am a man." Circle *a* is the self-order standing for sanitive and well disciplined life. Circle *b* is the self-disorder, standing for unsound and ill disciplined life.

My craving to live my sense of authority is the deepest need of my human being. Without insight, I can only seek for authority which I cannot recognize as mine. Every physician, clergyman, or educator of any kind is aware of his fellow man's dependence upon, and demand for, authority. It is hardly possible for a physician to absolve himself of living as if his patient could delegate authority to him. This most distressing circumstance of human living is rarely if ever recognized as such. It accounts for such dire needs in my human being as to be told what to do, to be helped by the strong one, to be rescued from helplessness, to be advised, counselled, persuaded, healed, or hallowed, by the proper "authority." *Along with any disowning of my authority must go my disowning of my responsibility.*

Now I am ready to state briefly the critical principle animating this work. *In my myth of infant helplessness I deceive myself most thoroughly and pay heavily for my inability to read the signs of this self-deception. At no time in my human life am I able to be more helpful than I am in my beginnings. During my intrauterine and first postnatal years I help myself completely. The idea of help, other than self-help, is incapable of physiological, biological, ontological, or any logical accounting. However, the myth of infant helplessness is glorified to such an extent that I expose it here maybe at great personal (including professional) risk. It is used to account for the equally mythological story that a mother not only can but must help her helpless baby. This first fairy tale prepares the way for my*

*teacher to live the imposture that he can educate his pupil,
and for my physician to live the illusion that he can cure or
help his patient in some way or another.*

*I pose the question: What difference does it make after
all if as a baby I grow my mother with her having, or not
having, the insight that she can help or harm herself only?
All of the advantage of truth hangs in the balance. If I
grow my mother with her having the insight that she can
help or harm herself only, I find this growth compatible
with my realizing that I can help or harm myself only. All
of my capacity for self-esteem is founded upon what realization I have that I am my own and only helper and harmer.
The health significance of this particular growth of self-
consciousness is inestimable. It is this conscious self-
knowledge which justifies and necessitates the writing of
this work. What kind of a specimen am I if I must consult
my somebody else as to whether I am in pain or not? Yet
I find each of my fellow men living his mind as if such a
meaning of consultation were not only possible but also
necessary.*

As I consider the sexual development of my human
being, I confront myself with its full measured nature. I
am a growth originating myself with female and male
elements, to wit, my mother and my father elements. As a
young male I grow all of my meanings for femininity and
masculinity. As a young female I grow all of my meanings
for femininity and masculinity. As each one, I create a
living of selfness most clearly describable in the form of
mental activity. As a little boy or little girl I grow the discovery of my own nominated sex and of my own nominated
opposite sex. As a man, if I grow myself to be incapable of

sensing my own femininity, then I must live a mentally dissociating kind of experience of my woman thereafter. When I marry, my talk about marital union being within must be only lip homage. The idea that my marriage is the opportunity for fuller living of my own masculinity and femininity will be a remotely inaccessible one which I cannot make the most of and enjoy the greatest self-advantage from. I am separating my idea of myself from my idea of everyone and everything else of my opposite sex, thus detracting from my appreciation of my greatness.

I exercise my wonderful organ, my eye, my ear, my sense of touch, but, as a rule, I am not able to live up to the wonderfulness and to the greatness of each. I, as consciously conceived, cannot own up to the marvelousness of my own human being, and therein lies a tremendous handicap. Who is there in my world, which I live in myself, who lives up to the wonderfulness of his human constitution? Whoever does, certainly conducts himself as a god. I grow my marriage. My awareness of my integration is not clouded by my home living, for I see myself as growing my family living. As my child consciously grows himself, he thereby aids himself in realizing his greatness. The inclusive and exclusive wonderfulness of human individuality is all that he can grow. A by-product of the healthy living of infanthood and childhood is the gradual becoming of healthy adulthood.

It is sickening just to take for granted that I exist. As I progressively uncover, and thus recover from, the habit deterioration of just taking my marvelous existence for granted, I experience all of the wonderful feelings analogous to the gradual restoration of sight where there was only blindness. The introduction into my life of the idea of self-help and its practice upgrade health, quite as inattention to this particular inspiration and drill downgrade health. Human life is for the purpose of living the true nature of mankind.

III. MY PERSONAL IDENTITY

All Nature is but Art unknown to thee;
All Chance, direction, which thou canst not see;
All Discord, harmony not understood;
All partial evil, universal Good;
And spite of Pride, in erring Reason's spite,
One truth is clear, Whatever is, is right.

ALEXANDER POPE

DURING decades of study and research in human nature I have noticed clearly that I, including my fellow man without exception, grow my studies of human life without seeing to it sufficiently that all of this study is observable as the growth of my own self. This kind of self-education, the kind not noted as human development, lacks the all important ingredient of self-consciousness. Self-consciousness is the *sine qua non* of self-health. Seeing all of my betweenness for what it really is and can only be, within-ness, is a process which is totally dependent upon progressing from self-unconscious living to self-conscious living. To use the figure of John Keats, everyone must, "like the spider, spin from his own inwards his own airy citadel." The enlightenment doctrine of *self-conscious individual independence* elevates the definition of every science in seeing each one for what it must be, a branch of the science of self. My own life must be the constant new creator of every fact of life. Such is the rule which governs all sane living, including research. Orthodoxy is healthful to the extent that it means living the life of conscious individuality. I enjoy all of the benefit of truthfulness to the extent that I can observe of myself, "I am an orthodox individual."

In this study of the science of self the term "self" is a synonym for whole person and means the inviolable oneness of human individuality. My specific purpose in using the all inclusive rubric "self" is to indicate that any one of my mental experiences which I do not entirely observe as exclusively my own is not observed truly. Such a self-deception (lie) is scientifically termed "repression." Self-deception unrecognized as such is the form of mental trouble which everyone suffers. Basically, it is the only form of mental illness. Montaigne recorded his sanity, "I look within myself, I am only concerned with myself, I reflect on myself, I examine myself, I take pleasure in myself."

Repeatedly I hear such a question as: "Why not use some other word than 'self'? Is not the term 'selfishness' generally considered to carry an offensive connotation? Why therefore deliberately invite antagonism by making the word 'self' the very key word to all of your meaning?" These well intentioned remonstrances and pleadings are themselves manifestations of self-aversion. More than any other word, "self" says definitely what needs to be said. The painful emotions mobilized particularly against recognizing its meaning attest clearly that truth. Homage to self-worship is not idolatrous. God *is* all. The principle of omnipresence is healthful. I hear the question asked, "Is it possible for me either to love or adore myself too much?" The answer is ever the same, "No, not at all. It appears possible, however, for me not to love or adore enough of myself." What I cannot see is the matter *of* me; that I can see is the matter *with* me.

Writing with self-consciousness involves a style which must seem wordy, if I have the habit of mind of writing as if I can be out of my mind. My reader must expect to find his reading of his *Science of Self* an adventure in new ways of self-expression, and accordingly, must be ready to start renouncing his need to live himself numbly in self-expressions clearly denoting self-unconsciousness. This ordeal, as every other ordeal of self-tolerance, is a mind healing and mind strengthening way of life.

The more I have addicted myself to self-ignoration the more irksome I must find the renunciation of that habit. In the writing of this book I have found it necessary to correct as many phases of it as possible, in order to bring it into line with self-conscious being. To begin with, I found it necessary to renounce the use of plurals such as "we," "they," "them."

May my enduring reader secure for himself the reassurance there is in it by imagining that his author too has had to suffer all of the pains involved in abstaining from his life long habit of self-disregard and its associated self-disesteem. May he also derive every possible satisfaction from growing the appreciation that his author has enjoyed from an access of health accompanying every access of self-consciousness. My health base of self-consciousness is my most cherished self-possession. Seeing myself as a complete, freely living individual is the only solid ground for any of my reality testing. All of my reality is of me, mine. My sensation and perception are, can be, nothing but the product of my current growing creativity. It is necessary for me as a conscious individual to renounce all such illusions as agreement with somebody else, accepted view, received opinion, authentic communication, and every such notion implying the myth of interaction.

"I object," speaks out my skeptical reader, "I object to your mode of communication which claims to be no communication. I presume you are an educator. If you neither see nor otherwise sense my between-ness, what is your theory as to how you get your meaning across to your fellowman? What about your profiting from the accumulations of wisdom transmitted to you from the ancients?"

Surely this is an objection calling for immediate and careful treatment. As Bacon described his self-grown learning, "I am the ancients." The educative process, that is, the way in which I learn, is no exception to my one fundamental life activity, by which I mean my self-growth. Each one of my sensations is a growing point of the very tip of my apical self. For instance, I learn my alphabet only by giving life to my teacher and then by my having him demonstrate his learning of his alphabet. Having thus developed this learning in a part of me (by having my teacher live it) the whole of me is thereby enlightened. The working of an unsolved puzzle is accomplished in the same way (that is, by growing equal to it). If I cannot work the puzzle, I give life to (create my own meaning for) one in my world who can. As I proceed to grow my puzzle solution, it is I (in this part of me I call my teacher) who is doing the puzzle. This new look at the learning process (as its being a partial self-activity enlivened by the whole learner) has two advantages. It furthers my proper self-appreciation of the truth that all help is self-help and advances my conscious opinion of my self-worth thereby guaranteeing my caring for myself properly.

When I find myself in trouble I find that what I am needing specifically to give myself is another dose of self-consciousness. Somewhat as my great physician, Thomas Browne, noted, "All existence has been but food for contemplation" and "We carry with us the wonders we seek without us." By living my life as if it is not mine, I practice self-amnesia, the source of mental disorder. It is not to my advantage to practice forgetting myself. The science of self (autology, self-psychology) is worthy of most careful consideration by everyone of my world. However, the very term "autism," or "autistic thinking," is, as a rule, most unfortunately misunderstood to mean mental abnormality. However, it really constitutes my withdrawn-from-the-world patient's one and only hold on his mental life. Withholding any part of myself from being appreciated as my own human being is a habit of my mind which I have come to see kindly, realizing that I first lived myself that way, as the only way in which I could at that time help myself. I have best access to the voluntary use of any part of my mind which I can live kindly. Now that I see that I can help myself by extending my self-consciousness to all of my living, I regard every stumbling block *in the way* as a potential and necessary stepping stone *on the way*. In other words, what I find habitually obstructive of my self-view is instructive for my true (full) comprehension of my wonderful HUMAN BEING.

It is divine to be human, quite as it is human to overlook the god's eye view. I have found that, in order to live myself sanely, self-consciously, I must make the effort involved. It might seem easier to live myself insanely, self-unconsciously, but that is only a seeming associated with my inability to discern, or interpret aright, the continuous protest of every organ of my physiology against such self-disrespect.

> They who reject the testimony of the self-evident truths will find nothing surer on which to build.
>
> ARISTOTLE

The only healthy living which anyone can long for is in the mind of man. The evolution to health which is needed and wanted begins at once with each person, a world unto himself, living the self-view: *I distinguish myself and live myself as myself. If I cannot develop myself at once to a high level of self-sincerity, I must have created some very real but unrecognized obstacles to my clearing the path of my progress in full life enjoyment. If I cannot at once discover what they are, I can be cheerful about my trying. In this life affirming attitude I feel my true existence. To live with self-consciousness is to cultivate freedom and to safeguard the development of all of my human power.*

I can certainly consider as self-evident my over-all truth: *I am all one.* A debate whether or not this expression of self-consciousness is economically shortened to "I" may be avoided by observing that "I am alone" sounds a little more lucid. I can get up absent-mindedly tomorrow morning or I can awaken and revel in the absolute certainty: I am myself unconditionally, absolutely and infinitely. Such is the awareness of self which insures full measured living. The peace that prevails with the arrival of the I identity is the product of equanimity, of self-repose.

It is impossible to live, or die, otherwise than as an individual. As my great American educator John Dewey once wrote: "The sensation gets significance, accordingly, just in the degree in which the mind puts itself into it. . . . That which is not thus idealized by the mind has no existence for intelligence. All knowledge is thus, in a certain sense, self-knowledge. Knowing is not the process by which ready-made objects impress themselves upon the mind but is the process by which self renders sensations significant by reading itself into them." Self-awareness adds sensitive humanness to the otherwise restricted view of one's self as consisting of carbon, hydrogen, oxygen, nitrogen, minerals and water. If I can employ my core of I consciousness, I thereby enable investment in my safe and sane world viewpoints. I can repose my I consciousness in the idea that I consist of heart, lung, kidney, stomach, brain and all such self-materials. I can repose my I consciousness in true self-views: I am a speck of dust. I am that drop of blood which was just in my veins. I am my wife. I am the criminal that was executed. I am a Russian. I am a fish. I am a tractor. I am ———, and I may fill in the blank with anything I please, including the unmentionable. There is no circumstance wherein, as a self-observer, I cannot helpfully repose my I consciousness and say: "This is what I am." Where I consciousness is, there is appreciated I geography, cherished I territory. It is precious health insurance to guard jealously the awareness of the personal necessity to be alone, all one.

Refusal to acknowledge that the exercising I *is consti-tuting and administering living* amounts to self-repudia-tion and accounts for the formation of self-amnesia. Where-ever I look, what I smell, what I hear, what I taste, etc.— if I consciously refuse to acknowledge any of it as an I experience, I may notice how I am attempting to disregard myself. Refusal to acknowledge, or even ignorance of, self-ness obstructs the self-freeing view: I consist of my uni-verse. Such refusal also clears the self-limiting view: I am an infinitesimal part of my infinite universe. The former is entirely self-respecting, the latter not.

As a physicist I assert: energy can neither be created nor destroyed. Literally translated this statement observes: something cannot derive from nothing; nothing cannot derive from something. I next consider this viewpoint in juxtaposition to the I-am reality. I can say accurately, "I am," but I cannot say with similar accuracy, "I-am was" or "I-am will be." I am is not the same as I was or I shall be. If I try to introduce anything to my attention but I-am, I am trying to deceive myself. By definition, saying, "I was" or "I shall be," rules out I-am consciousness. I-am *never was,* I-am never *will be,* I-am only *is.* The I-am self-evident truth discovers the problem of immortality to be a phantom problem.

If I could make a complete report on the I experience, it would be universal. It would be a merging sense of all-ness. There is no conceivable phase of my living where, as an observer, I cannot wisely and well repose in my I consciousness and say, "That too is what I am."

"Great Heavens!" exclaims my lively reader, "I presume you are still interested in me and in what I think of all of this I-am-the-many-in-the-one theory of yours. By the way, does not the biblical report of the revelation of Jehovah to Moses consist of the words "I am"? Isn't one definition of science that it is an exact language? If, as you claim, only I can help myself, you would make it a lot easier for me by getting out of this self rut of yours and talking the King's English."

Yes, it is recorded that Jehovah's words with his Moses were, "I am." In fact every magnanimous person in the history of my world has manifested his comprehensive self-consciousness in insightful self-observations. As to defining the terms I am using, for my present purpose the one indispensable definition of each of them is that it is a self-term, saying something about me only. This is a publication of myself, to myself, and for myself. Since I am in all of my living, my use of synonyms is unavoidable. Thus I may use "my life" to mean I am. As a mathematician, I may use one equivalent for another. Whether I say "I am" or "my mind," it is the same selfness of mine. My selfness, or creaturehood, in its particulars, is what I can be aware (certain) of. If I can live from the core of my mind consciousness, I can thereby repose my mind consciousness in my view that mind consists of living heart, lung, kidney, stomach, brain, son, daughter, neighbor, and all the rest of my universe. Further to exercise and thereby strengthen the idea: I can discover none of my living, of which, as a self-observer, I may not say, "That is what my mind is creating too." Of nothing which it senses, of nothing which it lives, can my mind wholesomely claim lack of identity.

Only where mind consciousness lives itself can the action of mind care be exercised. There is no possibility for my mind to have anything to do with anything which is not itself. It is the surveyor and the surveyed, the maker, the making and the made. To carry the point further, this perspective means my mind also creates my parent, my mate, and my offspring. My being includes my enemy. My mind includes my car and my fellow man's car. My mind includes my Napoleon. My mind includes my air. My mind includes my well wishes along with my ill wishes. My mind includes my denial that all is mind.

Seeing my personal identity in *all* that I live exercises my highest degree of mental power: self-consciousness. To illustrate: (My) De Quincey observed of one of (his) Wordsworth's utterances, "That is what I told you." Thereupon Wordsworth asserted his identity, "No: that is mine— mine, and not yours." Quite as my own Emerson observed, to quote a thought without a sense of authorship of it is tantamount to disowning one's own thinking capacity. Where I am incapable of sensing my personal identity in my living, there I indulge my illusion of being able to divide my life so that one part of me pretends the ability to exile the other.

IV. I INTEND TO ENJOY
GROWING MY HEALTHFULNESS

Nothing useless is and low;
Each thing in its place is best;
And what seems but idle show
Strengthens and supports the rest.

HENRY WADSWORTH LONGFELLOW

MUCH OF MY life may be lived with a part of myself sitting in judgment, as it were, upon the rest of myself, whimsically pronouncing one phase of my life "good" and another part "bad," one phase "important" and another part "trivial." The truth is that every element of it is wonderful, indispensable, and essentially my own vitality.

Acknowledged or not, I can be interested only in helping myself, the fullest acknowledgment of this self-interest being the high road to health. The recognition of my self-life, as being my only *possible* interest, is one of the major factors in mobilizing my self-forces for harmonious self-care. A most helpful motto is the following: I INTEND TO ENJOY MY HEALTH.

Any of my use of my word "selfish" in a disparaging (repressing) way is a case of the pot calling the kettle black, quite as this nihilistic trend is true of all detraction. I like to use the rubric "selfish," since it reveals to me, better than does any other word, my resistance to viewing my others as my own self-growths. The term means about the same as the word "egotistic," another instance of a precious meaning used mostly in a derogatory (repressing) sense. *It is essential for me to learn (grow) the self-view that the greatest egoistic autocrat is the one who studies and cares for the nature and needs of his world the most. Although it does not always harmonize with my mental attitude of the moment to ask myself to become more selfish in order to extend my charity with sincerity, nevertheless this is the direction in which I need to cultivate myself, if I will grow greater self-comprehension.* Acknowledged and cherished selfishness provides the only true altruistic habit of my mind. The very fact that this self-view may be terrifying to me reveals my powerful resistance towards developing my capacity for magnaminity.

I am wise when I begin to increase my insight regarding purposeful mental exertion and the benefit from my continued devotion to it. If I ask myself how to strengthen, and keep strong, my muscles, I say, "Practice such-and-such calisthenics regularly." And, if next day I observe: "Well I did the exercises outlined, so now what shall I do?" I would not hesitate to point out to myself the necessity for continuing the discipline. So it is with the development and maintenance of my mental strength. My clergy recognize the need for the *practice* of goodness. Let me recognize this need for the practice of healthfulness. I need to devote myself *consciously* to self-interest and self-care steadily and to resist every temptation to ignore it. There is nothing like acquiring self-uses that pay, while I am young, for solid self-help when I am young longer. It takes practice to learn the use of the self-curb and yet have range and freedom. I am wonderfully made in that I can learn, in time, to use as my ideal that which I once shunned as harmful: conscious self-development.

I heed that my everyone must appreciate his own individuality in the only degree possible, pending his helping himself to increase that truth feeling. As I mature I attend to continually increasing evidence of greatness in my human nature. I find that incentive other than self-benefit is false, in that it is impossible. I cannot set up a strange god before me, I cannot break my first commandment. I prefer to be virtuous since I cannot grow and develop well in any other way. I do not live in order to develop virtue. My living of it is my all. In my America, my government exists for me the citizen, I do not exist for the government.

I may easily demonstrate to my full satisfaction the all important truth that my essential over-all evaluation of my human nature is a happy one. For instance, if I consider my mental attitude of bitter resentment of somebody else's behavior to be solely and wholly constituted of my self-activity, my feeling of unhappiness immediately diminishes until finally I regard again my natural self-feeling of joy of living my truly wonderful human being.

By observing that all of my hurting is my own creation of it, I save vast energy which otherwise would be used up in complaining, protesting, blaming. Once I recognize that only *I* can hurt myself, I renounce complaining as obviously pointless, and the energy thereby saved is available for my healing process. What a saving!

Living Consciously

When not overwrought but quite at heartsease, my mind, thereby aware of its integration, does not mistreat its meanings for the inscrutable, the future life, the unknowable, immortality. The divinity of my self-identification in my *all that is* can be observed in my treatment of my meanings for "worms," "dust," and "pearly gates." All is equally heavenly and earthly. Life is more than interrogation and apostrophe; it is positively my all. The ultimate in affirmation is adoration, worship. Whatever is is adorable is a restatement of god is all. Such is the self-perspective which represents my most life affirming point of view. I designate it is as "the divine look," and it is ever a self-estimate. Fear of death holds no untoward meaning for me when I live right, in the sense of living with conscious self-devotion, but it is a common terror when I do not. This terror is a corrective sign, that is, a healthy homeostatic force.

As long as there remains one human being indulging blindly his wonderful capacity to imagine that he is not alone, there shall *properly* be crime, including fighting, in his world, as the helpful sign of his self-deception. Self-awareness and self-interest extending to all that I am never is the basis of illness, disease, fighting, war. Each of these painful ways is a wonderful sign telling me to mend my way. Thus, it is as if by my distressful living I automatically shout to myself to grow another way, a way which cultivates self-love leading to self-tolerance.

Growing my healthfulness necessitates my willingness to regard my consciousness of myself as being my most valued possession, which provides my development with all of the wisdom of life. With this insight I can identify my love of learning with my love of life.

I Intend to Enjoy Growing My Healthfulness

The whole hypothesis of school is on my own shoulders. I do not idle, or coast, or drift, into healthfulness. However, I do make myself healthful in the same instinctive way that I make myself hungry, or sleepy. Furthermore, my sense of identity in my feeling hungry, or sleepy, is the open secret accounting for my recognizing it as an imperative need of mine. Once I can similarly sense my identity in my various ways and means of making myself weak, or sick, then I am able to sense my imperative need to discipline myself to healthfulness.

V. SELF-AFFAIRS

If we call the sum total of sensory impressions "the sense world," we may state briefly that exact science issues from the experienced sense world. This sense world is that which, so to speak, furnishes science with the raw material for its labors.
However, this seems to be a very meager result. For the content of the sense world is, in any case, only something of a subjective character.

MAX PLANCK

EVERYTHING having to do with the activities which I call my sensation and my perception is entirely a matter of my own private business. My world is my self-begotten creation. My world outlook can be nothing but self-consideration. My precious possibility is to be wholly engrossed in my living of me. My very self-denial is self-indulgence. My disregard for my fellow man is the product of my restricted selfness. My selfness is my only possible motivation. My devotion to the enlargement of my selfishness, to consciousness of my world as my own, is a definition of healthful self-development. Self-sameness, my own personal identity, underlies my every meaning of otherness, of difference, of plurality. The only way I can live myself as truly outgoing is in the possibility that the direction of all my self-growth is from within out. My (illusional) unselfishness is fortunately lived as painful outlandishness. All of my outside is inside. With this kind of introduction I help myself to review my sensory growing for what it is —a self-development of mine.

My scientific reader here begs, "All of this way of thinking I have frequently heard classified as 'hot air.' Is it possible for you to be a little more concrete about these sensory growths by means of which you claim you develop your personality and attain your maturity? Please develop your thesis, of growing yourself as your sense organ grows, with a little more system. For instance, would it be possible for you to elucidate specific sense organ functioning and in that way demonstrate whether or not what is factually known about sensory physiology supports or undermines your allegedly 'scientific' conception of the allness of human individuality? Does not a searching analysis of your human mind necessitate some detailed study of your sense organs? For instance, how does my human personal eye grow its self-scenery, called 'vision' in the language I use? Or, How does that private living of my ear grow its self-sounds, called 'hearing' in my language, and so on?"

A more careful look at the nature of my sense experience may be helpful. Please note that where there is the most self-consciousness, there is the greatest humaneness and that the following discussion of my sensory living is undertaken at a certain risk of ignoring that it is all and only my *living* of it.

MY SEEING ME. Traditionally I call my eye "a receptor." In a similar misleading terminology I conventionally claim it is sensitive to a form of energy of wave lengths of about 397 to 723 millimicrons. When my wave length is less than 397 millimicrons I do not notice the ultraviolet color with the use of this receptor. Also, I do not notice the infra-red color or heat waves.

Within my range of visual sensitivity, I assert the illusion, "The distant stars may be reached." I offer myself the illusion, as truth, that my perception extends far out of myself through the deflections and refractions of millions of years. The outward path which this activity of my sense organ, my eye, *appears* to take, generates the breathtaking view that my appropriate system of reflectors could enable me to enjoy the sight of human behavior of my Inca civilization, or of my troop movements of every "World War" of history, and so on. In my already available coast-to-coast live television transmission, that which is already livable as history on my transmitter end is livable as current self-views on my receptor end. So-called human relationships cannot even be lived on the level of simultaneity. I can only live as my fellow man's history any perception or sensation of mind, which I refer to as "my fellow man." By the time I live my fellow man's voice his (my) expression of his voice is already a part of his past history. My Walt Whitman has poetized the self-ward living of his sensory perception:

> There was a child went forth every day;
> And the first object he look'd upon, that object he be-
> came; . . . .
> His own parents,

He that had father'd him, and she that conceiv'd him in
her womb, and birth'd him,
They gave this child more of themselves than that:
They gave him afterward every day—they became part of
him. . . .
The horizon's edge, the flying sea-crow, the fragrance of
salt marsh and shore mud;
These became part of that child who went forth every day,
and who now goes, and will always go forth every day.

I now continue my technical discussion of my eye and
other self-developments, heedful lest my scientific terminology either take for granted, or otherwise ignore, the
truth that my sensory living and everything about it is the
product of my own mental growth. Technically stated,
when I cling to the meaning of my sensory activities as
evidence of something other than myself, I thereby repress
the actual selfhood involved and then use the "return of
the repressed" disguised as not-self as the ground of my
faith in an external world.

I may now study, and note carefully, how my scientific
textbook and my other literature in one way and another
may appear as my attempt to carry my self-ignoration as
far as possible. My fixed idea of my science as being objective, impersonal, unselfish distorts my entirely personal
mental material so that I cannot recognize it as such (as
mine). Nothing can be the object of my mind except what
I alone personally experience (live). There can be no theory
of the constitution of matter (e.g., atomic or electronic),
which is not, first and last, a mental product itself.

The study of so-called "physiological changes" can be
nothing but a psychological performance. However, to
construct a theory of mind on the data of physiology *with-*

*out even recognizing each and every such datum as purely
mental itself*—well, Does such disorderly mental work de-
serve the nobly humble name of Science? Here is an anal-
ogy: Using my hand I model a hand of putty and then
proceed to study my model as my scientific procedure for
investigating the nature of my living hand! Than such
pseudo-science there can be no error more costly in principle or more cruel in practice.

*Any theory which attempts to bring the law of mental
life under the law of an unacknowledged but true product
of mental life must mislead from the very start.* Carbon,
hydrogen, oxygen, nitrogen—each is nothing but a mental
construct, as is any and every aspect of chemistry (including
biochemistry). The explanation of mind by means which
are nothing but ignored mind is an old story. The best way
for me to show that I have brains is not by cracking open
my skull against a stone wall. There is no antithesis between mind and matter, unless I succeed in forgetting completely that all of what I call "matter" is, and can be, nothing but mental matter, nothing but my very own mental
creation.

Here my reader, a student of the humanities, ventures
a comment. "I always thought that the brain motions and
the mental action are one and the same process viewed
from different vantage points. Thus, viewed from the physical or objective side the process is a brain motion; viewed
from the psychological or subjective side the process is a
mental activity. I like your attempts at accounting for *all*
of your meanings as being nothing but your mind's mode
of operation, for certainly that is the only possible humanizing process. I can see how you do not like to consider the

physiology of physiology, beginning as you do with your mind. Suppose you were a physiologist, or anatomist, or biochemist—what then? Do you deny that you are a material organism?"

With my earnestly humane reader I now gratefully observe that every kind of study of bodily and physiological meanings (somatology) is entirely a psychological event—study itself being nothing but psychological in its full extent from student to (his) study material.

My eye has many possibilities and limits as an organ of vision, such as size of the illuminated area, intensity of the light, duration of the exposure, region of the retina excited, and readiness of the retina. I have exploited each possibility and limitation in such a way that I may create a motion picture which lets me imagine that I am seeing figures in motion, although it is only my life which has any motion.

It is easier for me to see myself an entirely self-contained one, as I pass from (1) actually living the visual operation of seeing my automobile collision to (2) the visual operation of seeing my film of this kind of event, on to (3) my reviewing with my mind's eye the memory of my film depicting a collision. Through my television I create the conviction of seeing one or another part of my world event. With my stoboscope I may sense so-called motion as stationary. With my microscope I am able to grow the sight, and describe the configuration, of my diminutive sense organs, as well as I can describe the appearance of any gross part of my anatomy. My radar allows me to sense my object through my walls which are impenetrable for my vision.

In this discussion about the eye, I observe my illusion that my sensory living permits me to get out of myself, permits me to live something other than my own existence, for example, to see the stars. I note how the definite article "the" implies anonymity in general, and in this instance my not-self in particular. The most flagrant use of this repressing article "the" is in its use to call *my* world, *the* world.

I shall now proceed, paying more vigilant attention to my ignoring additional sensory data that are wholly and solely self-data. Every sign or symptom of disease, disorder, abnormality, or pathology is in truth a sign of health. Without such healthy signs denoting danger to my life, the possibility of recuperation would be eliminated.

A blind man suddenly gifted with sight is not able to discern magnitude distance or figures. My Voltaire cites the instance of his famous Cheselden, born blind in 1715, who by means of a surgical operation, at the age of fourteen, saw the light for the first time. He underwent the operation reluctantly as he was unable to conceive that the sense of sight could greatly augment his joy of living. The first use of his vision confirmed all that my Locke and Berkeley had foreseen. For a long time he could not distinguish dimension distance or form. All that he saw seemed to touch his eyes as objects of feeling seemed to touch his skin. Not until after two months experience could he discover that pictures represented existing bodies. It appears that one must learn to see quite as one must learn to speak or read. How very much an infant lives (learns)!

MY HEARING ME. As a growth center, misleadingly and consistently called "receptor" center, my hearing organ is so sensitive that the movement of one part of it by as much as a diameter of a hydrogen molecule may arouse my attention. If my native hearing growth were much greater than it is, I might develop an observation of the molecular movements of individual oxygen and nitrogen particles in my air. Actually, I notice in my hearing a vibration range in frequency of 16 to 20,000 vibrations per second. To be able to grow hearing above my frequency I would need to attain my dog's auditory development. The range of energy values (from just noticeable to the maximum) which I tolerate may extend from one to beyond 1,000,-000,000,000 energy units. My hearing growth device involves my electronic transmissions over my nerves; my specific auditory agent, in this instance, being my eighth nerve.

MY TOUCHING ME. My growth of sensibility known as "touch" creates my illusion of pressure deformity. Each touch organ is a microscopic end-organ, being in apposition with the end of a separate nerve fiber. Over a hairy region it is found on the windward side of sloping hair. Another touch end-organ is found elsewhere in my skin and still another resides deep in muscle. Whenever one of these growth centers creates sensation there emerges the feeling of touch, or of deep sensibility.

MY MOVING ME. If my foot moves without creating the sensation of touch, I am nevertheless able to state the direction and extent of movement. Thus, I can accurately assume a similar posture with the other limb. I may also place a window pane in front of my closed eyes, put my right index finger on one surface of the pane, and on the opposite surface place my left index finger in exact apposition to it.

I may perform another simple sense act by lifting in each hand an object of approximately the same weight. If the approximation is not too close I can observe which is heavier.

I also have a sense of posture and of station, as well as of deep sensibility. My sense organs which I grow and use for these purposes are localized in my deep tissues, such as muscles and tendons.

MY GROWING HOT AND COLD. My receptor with which I grow my function of discovering warmth is a loose ramification of nerve fibers located deep in my skin. I call each of these sense organs a "warm spot." The central part of the cornea of my eye has none of these. My forearm has one or two per square mm. In the growth of a sensation of warmth, the minimum effective energy is found to be 0.00015 gram calories per square centimeter per second lasting three seconds. Increasing degrees of heat are observable through my growing sensations of warmth until a temperature of 52°C is reached. With higher temperatures this organ destroys itself.

The growth of a heat sensation lives nothing but itself —even though my illusion holds that it reports the temperature of other objects. My block of wood and my block of metal of the same temperature do not seem to be equally warm. My metal frees its heat far more readily than does my wood, so that my sensation of heat in the former instance grows itself more readily. I can grow my sensation of heat *as if* it reports the heat of my object only when the temperature of my object varies from my body temperature. Otherwise I must assume that my body temperature represents the temperature of my object. If I have a fever I am able to report a consciousness of heat variation inaccessible to me if my body temperature is normal. If my temperature is elevated I establish a new range of consciousness of temperature variations. If in blushing I notice the sensation of warmth in association with blood circulating more freely through a given area of my skin, my contiguous warmth receptors are activated. By contrast, I may experience spasm of blood vessels, for instance in my fingers, and complain bitterly of lack of heat even in my warm room.

My sensory apparatus for appreciating cold temperatures finds itself more extensively distributed over my body than does that for the appreciation of warmth. I have about 250,000 separate cold spots, each of which I call my "Kraus end-bulb." At a temperature most habituated by my skin, that is between 27° and 32°C, I note cold most readily. However, at extremes of temperature, it ranges from difficult to impossible for me to discern accesses of cooling or warming temperature. On growing my sensations for my warm room, and next for my cold outside, my sensation of cold is at once appreciated but may be subordinated in a few minutes. As a rule my physiology text speaks of this kind of living continuum as "adaptation."

I can experiment with my three basins of water, *a, b* and

c; a is cold, *b* tepid, and *c* hot. My left hand immerses itself in warm water and my right hand in cold water for several minutes. Following withdrawal each hand grows its after image of warm or cold. I am conscious of each of these after images for several seconds. Then when each hand immerses itself in tepid water, I sense a new development of my warm right hand and my cool left hand. Above a temperature of 45°C I feel warmth as if cold. I must consider the possibility that my need for cooling becomes most intense and engenders my hallucination of cooling relief. This view may be added to existing ones accounting for paradoxical cold.

MY BALANCING ME. An ingenious device concerned with my sense of every kind of motion is located in my semicircular canal of my inner ear. Using it, the relative position in my space of each part of my body excites my awareness. I notice most readily acceleration or deceleration of my body in my space.

MY SMELLING ME. Inside of each of my nostrils is a two and one-half square centimeters area I call my nasal patch. Resident in each patch is the end-organ subserving the growth of the sensation of smell. Although this area is far enough up in my nostril to be largely inactive in my ordinary breathing it is readily excited by sniffing, as an act of smelling. My end-organ generating my sensation of smell is a microscopic rod-shaped structure yellow in color. Its surface end terminates in a hairlike process. My organ of smell grows the sensation of some 4,000 distinct odors called "flowery," "fruity," "spicy," "putrid" and "pungent." One part diluted with fifty billion parts of air can sometimes be detected with my sense of smell.

MY TASTING ME. My taste bud is found on my tongue, palate, pharynx, and larynx and anterior faucial pillars. With each taste growth a distinction is possible denoted as "sweet," "salt," "bitter," and "sour." With all growing at once, my taste blend is produced. Careful examination of my tongue reveals that it varies markedly in sensitivity in different areas as to the quality of the sensitivity grown. The tip of my tongue is most ready to grow the taste either of sweet or salty. Its lateral region most readily grows the sour or acid taste. Its base grows most readily the bitter taste. My taste organ is not found all over my tongue.

My taste organ grows its several sensations in a specific way, a way which corresponds with the molecular structure of my tasted object. An interesting biological discovery is observable in this process. For instance, if the molecular structure of my tasted object denoting sweetness is altered so that this structure takes on the mirrored image formation (of the sweetness molecular arrangement) I have another taste organ growing my sensation of bitterness.

MY GROWING MY HUNGER, THIRST, SATIETY, EVACUATION, RETENTION, ASSIMILATION. In addition to the discussion of each end-organ *as a mental power* might be added similar discussion of the growth of hunger, satiety, evacuation, retention, assimilation or any other sense development of such body living of my mind.

It has been found helpful by each of my several investigators to consider sensory impulses as electrical phenomena occurring in his nervous system. Thus, my sense organ relays the intensity of its sensory activity by the changes in rate of electrical discharge over my nerve. Weak sensory activity is associated with slow rates of discharge, while strong sensory activity is associated with rapid discharge rates.

The end-organ of my senses can be eliminated and I can deceive myself by believing that I am still using it, as for example, by hearing, seeing, and feeling. For instance, I close my eyes and press against their sides and notice the apparent sensation of color. The phantom limb is another illustration. Following amputation of my limb I may experience the feeling of pain which I locate in a distal portion of my limb, as if it were not amputated. Without clearer discernment I might decide that my limb should be disinterred and placed in a more comfortable position. It may be that the nerve formerly used for reporting sensations from that particular portion of the limb is now living in terms of scar tissues or other overgrowth. When I believe I can feel my painful foot, following its amputation, I am living an illusion. The accurate description of this illusion can only be given by me if I realize that, prior to its amputation, my foot pain was entirely a matter of my mental activity.

Each of my sensations may be, and consistently is, *imagined* as coming from outside in, as if light comes from the star, sound from the bell, cold from the ice, or smell from the air. Conventionally, I may say that my eye is stimulated by a biologically adequate external stimulus of the nature of light and that my every other sense organ is similarly activated by an external stimulus specific for it. The insuperable objection to this description of sensation is that it is not true to the life of my sensory organ.

MY HURTING ME. My end-organ growing (life-saving) pain is conceived to be a minute free nerve ending diffusely distributed throughout my body. However, no one who has tried to feel pain from a knife cut in certain areas of his brain has grown this sensation thereby. The pain sensation grows itself under conditions of extremes of heat and cold, electricity, pressure, chemical activity, and any like excess. My sensation of pain signalizes a threat of annihilation. In growing itself, this sensation is not well localized, tends to radiate, and has the quality of being unpleasant. At one time I imagined this sensation to be only the expression of overwhelming activity of every sense end-organ, no specific end-organ being required to produce it. Later observation disclosed the pain sense organ, revealing pain as an indispensable human aid. As an individual I grow my own unique capacity to endure and employ beneficially my ability to feel pain, including my painful feelings (guilt, hate, fear, jealousy, distrust, shame, and every kind of dislike).

Admittedly, it is helpful to treat of my human being in terms of physiology as a mental discipline. However, this present effort is in no sense aimed at being comprehensive in this respect, its one and only full intention being to treat my part-functions as individuations of my individuality. In other words, I sense the desirability of being mindful of my whole person as living its every particular. The more I have in mind my wholeness, the less I will tend to lose my sense of selfhood in the study of my parts.

I EXERCISE MY SENSE WORLD. My effort to develop a *right view* about any form of mental life properly begins with due appreciation that it is only and nothing but my mental life with which I am working. Thus, as far as my living of it is concerned, my personal experience of each sensation, or perception, is entirely my own living of it, in exactly the same sense that any other use of my mind is entirely my own living of it.

Fundamentally, it is necessary for me to be willing to live each sensation, or perception, which I do live. The fact that I live it (any sensation or perception) is *prima facie* evidence that I *wish* to live it. In this most basic sense of all, all of my living may be properly defined as "wishful living." In other words, if I do live any experience, rather than end my life with it, my very continuation of my living is proof positive that I prefer to live the experience rather than to end life on account of it. This preference, or choosing to live an experience, clearly implies wishful living.

Therefore, it helps me to be able to realize that every sensation or perception, which I experience, regardless of how painful it may be, is entirely and nothing but the wished for product of my own self-growth. My every sensation, or perception, originates and has all of its being in my own living of it.

This right view of my sensation, or perception, as being all and only an innate development of my life, all and only a native growth of my human constitution, is most essential for my right view of the integrity of my individuality. Thus, I would avoid the massive repression associated with my attributing my every meaning of externality to my ever increasing unconscious outer world complex. By continuously making myself unconscious through my repressed sensory and perceptual living, by such self-deception in my living selfness as not-selfness, I addict myself distressfully to an ever increasing habit of weakening and sickening my mind.

In my living my life, insofar as it is thus far possible, with a steady application to the extension of my consciousness of myself, I have made a profound searching study of the meaning of the idea, feeling, sensation, and perception of the definition of individuality, my individuality to be sure. I have discovered that my true appreciation of the allness of individuality has been gained only through my ability to recognize kindly, and thereby renounce cheerfully, resistance to such appreciation. Most helpful of all has been my discovery that I have been living my sensations and perceptions for the most part in the service of repression, tending to live each sensation or perception, as if it were a growth from without in (an impossibility), instead of as a growth of my own involving my extension of my own living (the only possibility). Much of my formal education and training in neurology and physiology has tended to favor my illusion that my sensory, and perceptual, experience is not entirely and only my personal living of it.

Observing that an illusion is an illusion is the only possible process of dispelling an illusion. My noticing that I live my every sensation, and perception, entirely as I live any other part of my existence insofar as I see it as nothing but an activity of my own individuality—this insight has liberated in me the vital energy essential for my being able to live my resistance, my illusion of opposition, kindly. I have been able to see that resistance is all and only about itself, about resistance: that my resisted living is all and only about itself, resisted living. Only the full appreciation of the individuality of each of my individuations has rescued me from living my life as if one part of me could be in conflict, any more than in agreement, with another part of me. *Conflict, quite as agreement, is an illusion based upon the delusion that one meaning can have something to do with another meaning.*

I submit that consciousness which is not lived as a personally felt experience subserves repression. I further submit that either sensation, or perception, which is not recognizable as being only and entirely the activity of a living self is also employed in the service of repression.

It is impossible for me to live other than as I please. It is possible for me to live myself as if I do not live as I please. Thus, if I live myself distressfully as in a serious accident, or a serious illness, it is only on account of the fact that it pleases me more to live myself thus distressfully than it would please me to end my life in order to successfully avoid such living.

It is possible to grow a habit of mind which favors my actual sensing of my identity at the same time that I am living my sensation or my perception. For instance, as I grow my perception of my you, it is possible for me to feel the authenticity of my living of this perception. My own living of my own you cannot be adequately described by the term "resemblance." "Identity" is the only word which describes self-sameness.

Can the data of psychology be anything but (individual) psychic activities? Is not all psychology self-psychology? Is not every possible meaning entirely a psychological construct? Is not all knowledge self-knowledge, either a conscious or unconscious plenitude of self-views? Is not individuality by definition unique, irreducible and autonomous?

VI. MY MIND'S PHYSICAL BODY

Whoever you are! you are he or she for whom the
earth is solid and liquid;
You are he or she for whom the sun and the moon
hang in the sky;
For none more than you are the present and the past;
For none more than you is immortality!
Each man to himself, and each woman to herself, is the
word of the past and present, and the word of
immortality:
No one can acquire for another—not one!
No one can grow for another—not one!

WALT WHITMAN

My HEALTHY free imagination appears to have no bounds, even showing itself able to posit bounds for itself, such as, "I can imagine only about myself," or "I can imagine also about my not-self," or "What I cannot live is thereby nothing." I cannot consider anything which is not my own consideration. To claim that I can do so is to fancy my ability to live beyond my means. I must live myself on "the outs" with what I have the *illusion* of experiencing as out of my mind. Simply by not seeing my greater or lesser mind as views of my own, I can deceive myself and claim that it is possible to produce a greater or lesser mind than my own. This exercise of constantly begging the question, as far as the use of my mind is concerned, strengthens my habit of self-deception. Even this exercise is a way in which I am helping myself as best I can, when I find it necessary to indulge it.

It is plain that all observation is self-observation; that when I talk about the perceptibility of matter, all I can in truth imply is that *that* perception is a living of my own human nature. However, if my habit of mind necessitates it, it is by means of my illusion of otherness that I may have to develop my mind, that I may require myself to extend my self-growth. First sight in the form of sensation or perception may be unrecognizable as (nothing but) self-evidence. Insight, which is self-consciousness, which is the feeling of personal identity, is recognizable only as self-evidence. Otherness as opposed to selfness introduces dualism, a devil's trap.

By "addiction to illusional otherness" I mean my habitual use of my precious illusional otherness without realizing its illusional nature, without seeing clearly that it is my own mental material. As an addict to illusional otherness, I must refuse to repose trust in myself as being able to live my external world and must complain that any scientist calling himself only a self-observer would have to leave out fundamental external facts. As an acknowledged self-observer I can, but do not have to, complain of my someone else in the first place, and beyond that I affirm my every illusion as a true self-reality (however illusional) of my own. In other words, as acknowledged self-observer I can also do what I can do as a declared self-ignorer. As a declared self-ignorer, however, I cannot do what I can do as acknowledged self-observer. For seeing which of two apparently conflicting claims, or views, is the true one, I have found it helpful to notice which one can subsume the other.

This degree of appreciation of self-consciousness appears to be as old as language itself. In Sanskrit, the ancient language of the Hindus, there is a word for it: *ahankara*. My *Webster's Dictionary* defines this term as follows: "The activity of making the subject (ego) an object, which is held to be the root of dualism and an illusion and ignorance of true being." Maxim Newmark also defines this term: " 'I-maker'; the principle generating the consciousness of one's ego or personal identity."

In his presidential address to the Royal Society November 30, 1859 Sir Benjamin Brodie spoke his mind: "Lastly, physical investigation more than any thing besides helps to teach us the actual value and right use of the Imagination—of that wondrous faculty, which, left to ramble uncontrolled, leads us astray into a wilderness of perplexities and errors, a land of mists and shadows; but which properly controlled by experience and reflection, becomes the noblest attribute of man: the source of poetic genius, the instrument of discovery in Science, without the aid of which Newton would never have invented fluxions, nor Davy have decomposed the earths and alkalies, nor would Columbus have found another continent."

John Tyndall, a most productive nineteenth century scientist who enjoyed the renown of his scientific world, observed, "The reading of the works of two men, neither of them imbued with the spirit of modern science, neither of them, indeed, friendly to that spirit, has placed me here to-day. These men are the English Carlyle and the American Emerson. To Carlyle and Emerson I ought to add Fichte, the greatest representative of pure idealism. These three unscientific men made me a practical scientific worker."

My self-composed questioning implies my readiness to grow myself in the direction of my questioning. At this juncture my reader may ask, "Will you please put into words your mind's view of the mind-*versus*-matter problem, a subject which has been the source of much puzzlement for me. Or better, can you draw a picture which will clarify the location of body and mind, as you see it? I am conscious that I have a body. I suppose that means that my mind can live meanings of a body category. Here I begin to find myself answering my own question."

First things first. If one of my colleagues, an anatomist, should say to me, "You certainly believe that the mind is resident somewhere in the nervous system, don't you?" my considered reply might well be: "That is an excellent *idea.*" Simply by my colleague's reminding himself (through the term "idea") that all of his anatomical data are nothing but psychological data, to begin with, he thereby avoids the possibility of forgetting that his mind always creates its own anatomy, physiology, biochemistry or physics. Although for convenience I sometimes divide my psychology into pure psychology (by which I mean the psychology of acknowledged psychology) and applied psychology (by which I mean the psychology of unacknowledged psychology, for instance, anatomy), nevertheless there can be really no applied psychology any more than there can be really any applied science.

All of the distinction of sanity lies in the view, the physical body of my mind; all of the distinction of mental

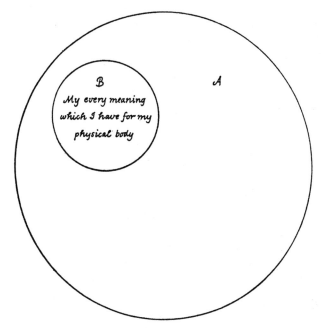

CHART II. *My Mind's Physical Body*
Circle A. My view of my mind
Circle B. My view of my body

disorder lies in the view, the mind of my physical body (brain, central nervous system, or "physical being").

Again, this kind of comprehensive appreciation of mental vitality has been beautifully pictured by my ancient

(ever present) Plato: "As I proceeded I found my philosopher altogether forsaking mind or any other principle of
order and having recourse to air and ether, and water,
and other eccentricities. I might compare him to a person
who began by maintaining generally that mind is the
cause of the actions of Socrates, but who, when he en-
deavored to explain the cause of my several actions in
detail, went on to show that I sit here because my body is
made up of bones and muscles; and the bones he would say
are hard and have ligaments which divide them, and the
muscles are elastic, and they cover the bones, which have
also a covering or environment of flesh and skin which con-
tains them; and as the bones are lifted at their joints by
the contraction or relaxation of the muscles, I am able to
bend my limbs, and this is why I am sitting here in a curved
posture; that is what he would say, and he would have
a similar explanation of my talking to you, which he
would attribute to sound, and air, and hearing, and he
would assign ten thousand other causes of the same sort,
forgetting to mention the true cause, which is that the
Athenians have thought fit to condemn me, and accordingly I have thought it better and more right to remain
here and undergo my sentence; for I am inclined to
think that these muscles and bones of mine would have
gone off to Megara or Boeotia—by the dog of Egypt they
would, if they had been guided by their own idea of what
was best, and if I had not chosen as the better and nobler
part, instead of playing truant and running away, to
undergo any punishment which the State inflicts."

VII. THE PRACTICALITY OF MY SELF-CONSCIOUSNESS

Let the incommunicable objects of nature and the metaphysical isolation of man teach us independence.

EMERSON

MY ILLUSION of an external world (separate from me) has enabled me to create the name "objectiveness" as opposed to "subjectiveness." Using illusioned objectiveness, I feign to see things as they are. This self-imposture, objectiveness, may seem to me to serve self-interest, whereas subjectiveness (my true posture of self-revelation) may not. However, a great minded person may be aware of observing self only. His comments begin with a stated, or implied, "May I ask you to consider," "As I see it," "In my opinion," "From my viewpoint," "It seems to me," or, "For me it is this way." The acknowledged great man is committed to interest in *what is,* and for that reason considers *himself* only.

Often I find directly mentioned, or alluded to, difficulties in attaining objectivity, quite as if objectivity were at all possible. A real problem is the neglect of the fact of the absolute impossibility of anyone's describing any other person or thing but himself. The work which deals wholly and solely with such truth will accomplish the most for mankind. Blind insistence that it is possible to be objective is thoroughly understandable in terms of one's compelling need to disown his mental material and compensate by using it without feeling responsible for it.

I have a concept of being practical. What is practical except what furthers the conscious practice of myself, self-practice? Nothing. Is it practical for me to live as if I can lose my mind? Is it practical for me to consider my mind dissociated into self and not-self, without my realizing that my not-self is, and can be, only unacknowledged self? I may profitably grow the kind of insight that my religious fellow man has grown: Everybody has to save his own soul; somebody else cannot do it for him. As I have already recorded, costly teaching that I have created of my selfness is my unrelieved *illusion that one person can do something for or to somebody else.* Of all the weak teachings of human being, that is a contender for first place.

Let me contemplate for a moment the therapeutic value of being close to nature. I create an environment for myself by means of which I can easily recognize that all of my living is personal. Perhaps this is my growing my farm, or my woods, or my cottage by the lake, or my mountains, or my beautiful garden, or my wide open spaces. Wittingly growing my environment, I am refreshed. My own (acknowledged) fresh air is uniquely healthful. Here is my (self) medium for my growth of sanity. Here I see and recognize my order in my nature. I have the feeling of its being a part of me, and thus easily approach the truth that it *is* mine. I may say that the world is in chaos, but that is an illusion. *My* world that lives in me is in perfect order, exactly as it is. But my mind gets into apparent disorder through my inability to acknowledge that what is, what truly *is*, is my self. Where my nature is lived consciously as farm, woods, cottage, lake, mountain, or garden, I am forced to see and acknowledge order. I never observe my tree, or my stone, confusing itself with another tree, or another stone. In nature loving, I live easily the truth of my true nature. My trees or brushes, my bushes or flowers, are instances of honest struggle for self-survival. My life finds it profitable to live appreciatively its natural phenomena, and thus feel itself in harmonious accord. My world is in exactly the order I ordain. Tomorrow my sun will probably be on time. I can feel very secure about my Big Dipper and Southern Cross, my river flowing, and my tide coming and going inexorably. It is no gain to defy, and so profitable to deify, my circumstances of my necessity.

Unawareness of the following truth does not alter it. *No man is free to misbehave in any way.* My human constitution is so constructed that a loss to my anyone is a loss to me, a gain to my anyone a gain to me. The true definition of loss or gain for me must be described in terms of my own constitutional necessity to live both loser and gainer. I am bound to take care of my living of my universe, as it is a part of my own life. Only unawareness of this truth accounts for all of my short-sighted (illusion of) human relationships. I cannot lie to myself about the exclusively personal meaning of my externalities and remain healthy. The more awareness there is of my human integration, the more I have developed appreciation of the necessities of my total world. Justice for my all, is a necessary ideal to uphold my every person's constitutional order. Health to all of me is a necessary ideal to uphold my every person's constitutional normalcy. Devotion to all of me is a necessary ideal to avoid my every person's constitutional neglect. Most desirable is it that my insight cover the entire scope of my human nature. I cannot neglect my self with impunity.

If I exercise blindly my illusion of others, I cease to operate on the level of sensing that one man's loss is another man's loss, and one man's gain is another man's gain. I do then begin to operate on the archaic level of sensing that one man's loss can mean another man's gain, and one man's gain can mean another man's loss. In such self-ignoration I overlook this truth: since each personified individuation of me which I live as my fellow man is a world to himself, my greatest concern might be that of extending as fully as possible my feeling of kindness, since my all is my kind. I love my neighbor as myself, for in every possible sense as far as I am concerned, (my) he is lived by me.

A gain to one man is a gain to all.

A loss to one man is a loss to all.

No man can lose from another's gain.

No man can gain from another's loss.

For me to grow my fellow individual who must hurt himself unprofitably is to live my fellow man helping himself but shortsightedly. If I deem myself ill, my shortcoming consists in my being unable to extend my attention to the fact of my existing greatness, to the nobility inherent in my human nature, to my truly wonderful claim to reverence as divine, to my feeling of perfect equality with my own *human individuality*. I am fortunate if I can learn that there is no feelingless humanity, that all life is passionate. The circulation of love throughout all of my personal life (human being), a health necessity analogous to the circulation of the blood throughout my body part of me, is the chief concern of health.

When I pass out of self-blind into self-perceiving living, my sense of mental enlargement is so pleasing that it even may distract me from staking my claim upon its source, of patenting the process (of making myself conscious) to operate for my continuing benefit. Progress in recognition of self, with ever diminishing apparent unself, is the account of the attaining of any one's civilization worthy of the name. Pending this specific kind of individual development, each one of my mankind must suffer the goads helpful to finding self-conscious living. Infatuation with my apparent not-self of sun, moon, stars, and earthly wonders, is a costly conceit. When I do not know what I stand for, I may fall for anything.

Only a mind that practices awareness of its integration can have access to the good-natured kindness which makes allowance for whatever might be, which can sense the self-benefit in either a justice for all or love-thine-enemies or love-thy-neighbor-as-thyself viewpoint. To renounce one's more constricted self-interests for broader selfish claims (for one's others) is to indulge and enjoy the essence of one's kindness which binds selfness with love, with adoration. Allegiance to all of self is the right (adequate) incentive to duty, decency, fidelity, humility, and morality of all description. Every man is his own wonderful end, and whom he meets with in life is *his* own wonderful end.

VIII. I CREATE MY OWN
EXTERNAL WORLD

High walls and huge the body may confine,
And iron gates obstruct the prisoner's gaze,
And massive bolts may baffle his design,
And vigilant keepers watch his devious ways;
Yet scorns the immortal mind this base control:
No chains can bind it, and no cell enclose;
Swifter than light it flies from pole to pole,
And in a flash from earth to Heaven it goes.
It leaps from mount to mount; from vale to vale
It wanders, plucking honeyed fruits and flowers;
It visits home, to hear the household tale,
Or in sweet converse pass the joyous hours;
'Tis up before the sun, roaming afar,
And in its watches wearies every star.

WILLIAM LLOYD GARRISON

I AM MY own outside of me. I live all sides including my
outside. I cannot count myself out. I take sides, all sides.
My sensory living is one side of me. My perceptual living
is another side of me. All of my scientific living is my own
human growth.

For the important purpose of upholding awareness of mental integration it is necessary to realize that I grow my sensation and perception as I grow all of me, *from within out*. My sense organ is my means of extending myself as a being. By means of my sense organ I may create the *illusion* of uniting two parts of me rather than create the helpful awareness that I am only extending, enlarging, my oneness. One such illusional uniting part would be my acknowledged self, and the other my acknowledged not-self. By means of my sensory growth, I develop my *alleged* external world which really is entirely my own internal creation.

All I can do ever and everywhere is live my here and now. I can pretend to be a time server and a space server and must live that pretense to the extent that I claim to live in my world, not seeing clearly that my world must live in me. All of my meaning for motion is my life's activity; for space is my resistance to my ever present here; for time is my resistance to my ever present now. My consciousness is not the same at any two stages of my development. There is nothing old in my life or under my sun. All of my living is novel living. My consciousness of my past consciousness is not my past consciousness. Memory is an illusion. The claim to be able to relive my past life is no more valid than my claim to be able to foretell my future. My awareness of my past awareness is not that past awareness itself. Yesterday's awareness cannot be relived. May I be aware of living the only life there is to live, *now* and *here* living.

Acknowledgment that all of my mental living material, including each sensation and perception, is subjective (entirely personal) is a restatement of my familiar work of making self-conscious what was once self-unconscious. There is no poorer health prognosis than that expressed in the claim to be able to get at external data. Such mental orientation means that my imagination is stuck at the mental level of sensation and perception, wildly imagining such living to be non-mental. In evaluating *any* of my living as not mine alone, I thereby forget myself, create an amnesia for that part of my identity, and thus weaken my mind. Distressing awareness of my weakness helps me to strive for strength.

Most likely the first consideration which I make, as I begin to study (grow) insights such as the illusion called "external matter," or "the evidence of my senses is only self-evidence," is that I ought not to have my wonderful facility falsify my human being. The apparent perception of external matter is really a valuable facility, for it always does service for lacking insight. In the sense that it compensates for inadequate self-consciousness, it may be designated specifically as a most useful illusion. It may be a person's only means of preserving his life. The word "illusion" popularly has a bad name, and that in itself may tell me much, rejection being an important first sign of acceptance. Any and every meaning has all to do with my mind. There cannot be something apart from my mind. Even the claim that I can enjoy life other than my own is itself a work of my mind, compensating for my lack of realization that my all is mine. By recognizing apparent externality as a part of my mind, I can deal with it directly. By regarding apparent externality as *other than my mind*, I have to introduce mental dissociation to help myself and thereby forfeit the health-giving orientation of the awareness of my integration. My mind helpfully aware of its integration recognizes itself as a homogeneous unity.

Each progressive step in my self-consciousness is made with my feeling ill at ease until it is fully achieved. Once lived through, however, I lose the sense of feeling ill at ease and instead enjoy an access of self-esteem corresponding with the fact of my self-insight. Suppose I cannot realize that my soul, or mind, is my own and that all I live is an animation of the soul of me. Suppose I do not have this power to observe every property of my individuality in each one of my individuations. In other words, suppose that I do not have the mental strength for observing that my mind provides not only the subject matter but also the object matter of my perceptual living, quite as it does the subject and object matter of my other imaginings.

To illustrate, I grow the perception of my car in motion in such a way that I shall find myself injuring myself by the living I call "being run down." I can escape this living of injury with the greatest economy by recognizing it entirely as the growing of two meaningful self-views, one a perception representing my individuation called "oncoming motor car," the other a conception of my whole self as a potential victim. Less economically, I might have to designate my actual perception, oncoming motor car, as a necessary illusion and thereby save myself injury. Still less economically, I may avoid accident by living the (unrecognized) illusion that my individuation "motor car" is nothing but externality. Of these three ways to save my life, the least used one in my world is the most economical of them all.

Who in my world does not indulge his illusional living

without seeing that he is thereby confirming a habit of self-deception? The immediate life saving necessity is that I escape having myself run over. Certainly it is to my advantage to escape by using my illusion of external oncoming motor car, if I cannot escape simply by seeing that my perception oncoming motor car is a living of my own perception.

Suppose all I have is the mental strength to view my living my sensation as no different from living my other imaginings. In such a predicament I might say to myself that I do not like the sensory illusion of being on a precipice and, therefore, distract myself with a more pleasant view such as, abyss means nothing to me. The truth is that I must live myself in one distinct way when I imagine my sensing, or perceiving, and in another distinct way when I imagine without creating sensation or perception. I would not live long if I were incapable of distinguishing my living my perception and my living my other imaginings. Without the capacity for this distinction I would not grow the life saving negotiation and other life affirmation associated with my sensory living. *The perceptual part of my living is very extensive, so that my ability to be conscious of it as entirely my own living is an absolute health requirement.*

I now consider my mental activity, which I ordinarily call "a worm" and accurately discover that my worm can consult only his own living powers for wriggling about, even though he appears to recognize the difference between his rock and his loam. My worm is self-contained and as such can have nothing to do with my rock or my loam. I certainly wonder about the evolution of my mind, including how each of my living creatures is integrated in this respect. My Mr. Worm certainly can not accurately claim to be feeling the rock. He can only feel himself. If he just grows and goes pushing ahead, so to speak, he may be finding himself obstructing his own progress by means of his rock.

I consider the statement "one communicates with another" or "something passes between one and another." Then I consider what is possible, and see that what I mean by "between" must be within. Thus the illusion of communication dispels itself. I may cherish my illusion of communication as a kind of unsevered umbilical cord. There is no communication between minds, or between parts of a given mind, but my wonderful imagination can claim that there is.

Full measured individuality permits the most accurate usage of helpful mathematics, of such formulae as universal constants, of such scientific strategies as triangulation and similar scientific means. Seeing my world as mine involves no loss of any kind, other than the loss of my unrecognized self-deception. In my world every one of my human beings lives his 3.1416 in as uniquely individualistic a way as he lives any other part of his human being, for instance his hand.

My own life appreciation is the master principle of my education. I have discovered that *all* teaching founded upon the illusion of communication is pedantry. Individuality excludes externalization. Life can experience itself only, can not externalize itself. In whatever direction of my existence I delude myself with my illusion of communication—right there I forego my conscious sensibility.

"Do what I say," "Do as you are told," "Pay attention to me," "I'll show you how," and all such expressions which vainly attempt to support an illusion of significant externality, at the same time develop in their users an illusion of insignificant human being. Every day I test the worth of this theory (that all of my externality is nothing but my own life's creation), and every day I grow evidence of its indispensable value for developing my life safely, sanely, and satisfyingly.

IX. GROWING MY EXTERNAL
WORLD SELF-CONSCIOUSLY

It is easy in the world to live after the world's opinion;
it is easy in solitude to live after our own; but the great
man is he who, in the midst of the crowd, keeps with per-
fect sweetness the independence of solitude.

EMERSON

As an infant, am I able to evaluate accurately the personal growth meaning of my sensory activity? I lean to the view that I live *me* and only me, unquestionably and unquestioningly, as infant, and in no sense distract my sense of being with philosophical or psychological repudiations of being. I study myself as a baby, and just see eager living. My life sequence begins and ends with self and lives all pluralism as its own.

Consider a life episode depicting the results of efforts at self-ignoration. Once upon a time I had my Italian Naples rocked with laughter by the comical antics of my clown Carline. About that time I had one of my fellow men racked with crying over his unhappy life. He consulted his physician about his depression. His physician prescribed,

"Go see Carline, he makes everyone laugh." My fellow man replied abjectly, "I am Carline."

A story of the use of insight in industry, a local story of my human being's wheels, highlights the practical importance of insight about self-consciousness. My automobile manufacturer canvassed his prospective automobile owner to investigate demand. Thus he asked: "What kind of a car would you like to own?" The response he received consistently emphasized the economical, the practical, the unadorned, the simple. "I want low cost, no trimmings, safe and simple transportation." With this restricting research-finding my automobile manufacturer deemed it advisable to use a different approach. So he asked, "What kind of a car do you think your neighbor would like to have?" Here imagination enlivened the response, which consistently scored the high-powered, much-accessoried, costly pleasure wagon for seeing America first. I may live myself in my neighbor freely while I am otherwise holding myself down.

Accepting the meaning of mind as self-function, my mind will do what it must and can. One of its facilities is self-consciousness, mind sight, self-observation. It pays me to observe my being, of which my doing is a part. Effective attempts to regulate my functioning will include observing, recognizing, negotiating my mind's agencies which I recognize as its activities. In other words, all I can ever do is live, exercise my mind. There can be no self-ignoration. That is obviously an impossibility. There can be the illusion of self-ignoration and vain efforts to achieve self-ignoration. That is the obvious, and only, possibility for my self-producing the disesteem which, adequately interpreted, enables me to start crediting myself as being the creator of my every creation.

It is a necessary condition of my human nature to be, and hence express, all that characterizes my humanity. Being *it* is expressing it, and it is to my advantage to grow myself with a complete self-feeling. To deny the existence of whatever is is self-repudiation, for it is my whatever is. However, to the extent that my mind is undisciplined with self-consciousness, I must disown and consider as alien expressed parts of my human being which I may designate as "elseness," "otherness," "not-I," "not-self," "you," "they," "he," "she," or "it." Thus I may speak insensitively of extrinsic factors operating upon me, thereby succeeding in losing sight of my inclusiveness and non-exclusiveness. When I am unable to accept, recognize as my own, the misbehavior of my others, my aggressive rejections spare me consciousness of guilt feelings. My active avoidance of any aspect of living is avoidance of true but thus disowned and disarranged meanings of myself. Such self-unconsciousness comprises all incivism and every other form of "insanity." * As each unwelcome (self) meaning develops itself I protect the limits of my acknowledged self with the screening device, "This pleasantness is I," but "That unpleasantness is not I." The route out of this rut is for me to see clearly, adorably, its use as a temporary defense against my attempting awareness of immediately overwhelming conscious self-tension. It is a gain for me to be able to go (grow) unconscious, whenever I cannot bear (be aware of) an insufferable necessity of my living. However, following such a numbing experience, I may later

* A technical medico-legal term.

grow the mental strength required for seeing it clearly as all my own living of it. Such is my process of mental healing.

Every one of my human beings lives his own particular hermit's existence. My everyone lives in a restricted zone, with devastating forces all a part of him. (My) each one plots out his own world reservation, living a voluntary imprisonment thereby. From the bountifulness of my human nature I select and virtually claim: *"This* is my reservation, and while *that* is a part of me too, I shall not claim it for now." The overwhelming nature of my universe is never clearly observed for what I actually have it to be. After I set up my safety zone I like to ignore what I have before ignored. Meanwhile, I prefer to *imagine* that I am respecting all of my human being. Thus I slip easily into talk about accidents and external necessities of all kinds, for I consider such to be impersonal. (My) every man, regardless of his awareness of his mind's integration, sets up limits of conscious self-operation in his new self-developments. He extends these limits at the risk of feeling overwhelmed, at the risk of losing his sense of identity.

"Can't you see you're mistaken?" interposes my reader. "Can't you see that you are dehumanizing your dearest, as well as every other one, by denying that she, or he, exists apart from you? Don't you notice that you defeat your very purpose of being kind, humane, or even civic, by disposing of all your human relationships summarily as nothing but so much living of your own? Don't you have enough love to be able to share? Are you so short on love that you cannot provide for the existence of your own mother, or father? Maybe if you ask yourself such questions as these you might come to your own senses, and leave other people to theirs. At least own up to the fact that you don't know if there is anyone or anything but yourself. Even the introspectionist Berkeley acknowledged that much (other-than-self love)!"

Yes, my very own loving and lovable reader. Yes, I am able to regard myself as mistaken in every way. Yes, I am even able to produce my own view that I cannot be sure that there is no one but me to live me, that I cannot be sure that my externality does not exist separately and apart from my living of it all. And where do I find myself after all of that exertion? Where do I find myself after noticing my living the view that my dearest love is no part of my living at all? Where indeed, but back to the fact of my own self-living which I started from with the deliberate intention of escaping! All of such living of ideas, views, feelings, sensations, perceptions, and what not, *can only serve to demonstrate my one and only truth: my life!* What else? What else? Oh, *that* else? Must I not live *it*, that is, *be* it, for my it to have any and every possible meaning for me? Yes, I can think of my human relationships and see the meaning of the word "relationships" as being a useful patch upon wounded human individuality.

If I could draw a line between what I call one individual and what I call another, what is the nature of the relationship? Evidently there is none. *Individuality cannot be relational.* Human life is a matter of every man his all for himself. When I say that I am doing something for someone else, I am both ignorant and untruthful. How can I have an unselfish act, or thought? I cannot jump out of my skin, leave my senses, go out of my mind. I am all there. "Here I am, and there you are" needs to be recognized as the perpetuation of falsehood and stated accurately: "Here I am and there I am also." All of my immaturity and all of my mental illness is reducible to my calling myself somebody else or something else and to my illusion that anything foreign to me can have anything to do with me. My friend often expects to do something for somebody else. It is helpful for him to discover such perpetuation of self-deception. My patient who is aware of his integration is no longer claiming that his doctor cures him, for he is seeing more clearly the self-limits of all of his activities. Whatever selfishness exists is always wonderful and really the only foundation of all that goes under the name of humanity. Whatever is termed "unselfishness" is the only foundation of all that goes under the name of inhumanity. However, even unselfishness is primitive humanity. When I act in a narrow appreciation of my selfhood there is room for me to extend my appreciation of my selfishness, in my Coleridge's famous phrase, to grow "enlightened selfishness" from the realization that narrow selfishness does not provide complete coverage of myself.

Every pretense of departure from my self-order is attended by a constriction of my observation of my human nature's all inclusive meaning and thereby a diminution in sensing my self-esteem. My best is found in me, not in a not-self nowhere! Where is nowhere? The illusion of self-detachment is the one sign of immaturity and of illness. There is only one way for me to see to it that I become great, that one way is by observing the greatness I have grown. Who can claim the sun, moon, and stars as his very own and not sense the true grandeur of his magnificent being! This function of full self-measure is the office of full consciousness. *Consciousness is the being of awareness of being.* Ambition to be great, the ruling error of my weak mind, is my alternative for observing my greatness. Full self-development entails devotion to growing myself with ever present appreciation that my growth is wholly and solely my own. When I am "wise to myself," I am the exponent of conscious self-development. The more I accept the nature of my total solitude, of my unique being, of my all inclusive oneness, the nearer I can approximate an accurate description of my other one individual, animate or inanimate.

My reader may ask: "Can you adduce any striking proof that the propensions of every human being, not just of yourself, include this strengthening, healing, and in every way understandably happifying property called by you, inviolable individuality? The rest of us in the world cannot, too! Our dictatorial we is far more powerful than your sovereign I. Life to you is composed of one portion, yours!"

Yes, I have found that my living of myself heterogeneously has had too many disadvantages springing from the signs of my living myself carelessly thereby. I can write only of, to, by, and for myself. I am thus doing all I can possibly do to see to it that my own dear reader sees how he has had his writer help himself. True, I frequently write as if I could be writing for a somebody else not my own. Therein *is* dire confusion. I find myself again and again living my own self-grown fellow being, quite *as if* that being has a separate existence, apart from mine. For instance, I grow the view described loosely as "looking at a sunset." Although this picture is entirely my own creation, I may live it as if it had a creator apart from myself, *as if it is not my own creation.* Thankfully, I may grow subsequently the view that my idea of a separate creator is, after all, also entirely my own creation. This after thought is a conscious self-recovery and as such is lived along with an access of self-esteem. *I cannot view myself in all of my wonderfulness and protest or complain about any shortcomings.* Treating myself with the true view that sanity consists in living my instinct along with my insight may be overwhelming. I may illustrate this viewpoint by considering the oneness of my contempt. Due to a corruption of my language, which in itself is the expression of the corruption of my mind, I may say, "I am contemptuous *of* somebody or *of* something." This implies that one thing can have something to do with another; namely, that contempt can have something to do with something or somebody, whereas contempt can be only and all about contempt, itself. Every mental activity can only have to do with itself. *An individual consists only and all of individuality; hence, every element of my being consists entirely of its own individuality.*

Contempt is entirely of, by, about and for contempt. If the pretense is lived that this oneness can be violated, then the fact of living pretense is heralded by some sign or symptom of oppressed truth. There is no possibility that one thing can have anything to do with anything else. Despite all of the appearances to the contrary, a chair is a chair consisting entirely of nothing but its own chairness. I try to add anything but chairness to a chair and I am no longer true, except in so far as my pretense is a true pretense. Being happy about something; being sad about something; being glad, or guilty, or angry about something —each is an accurately inaccurate observation. It is truly an untruth. Negation always cancels itself. Stated in another way, negation is always an affirmation. I must affirm a negation in order for it to be.

My reader's mind now voices itself pleasantly, "How you can dilate on your favorite subject! How did you develop your ability to say the same thing over and over, 'self-conscious living'? As I review what I have already read— or, as you would say, 'as I live over my already lived reading'—I notice that you have not been able to clear your writing of my charge that it is, itself, an effort on your part to communicate your superior wisdom to an inferior external world. In other words, if your intention is to create your external reader as being entirely your own, it will pay you to work harder at it."

I see that more clearly now. And my seeing it is what I need in order that I may make my further writing reveal more clearly my avowed intention to dilate upon my one and only kind of help: self-help. I have applied myself consciously to this specific kind of work now for years, so that my writing has that experience in it. Whoever (of my world) will try to speak or write without thereby creating the illusion that he can externalize himself will realize the difficulty in this undertaking.

X. W-H-A-T ABOUT ME?

*Ever strive for the whole; and if no whole thou canst
    make thee,*
Join, then, thyself to some whole, as a subservient limb!
Let none resemble another; let each resemble the highest!
How can that happen? let each be all complete in itself.

SCHILLER

TWO PRINCIPAL views underlie *Living Consciously: The Science of Self.* One portrays the fact that everyone of my world already enjoys a certain development of his self-enlightenment. The other pictures the truth that everyone's extent of self-consciousness is not a fixed or predestined degree; that it is not only possible but most desirable for everyone to devote himself to the life work of extending his self-consciousness.

My being is any and every meaning which I live. Meaning is all that can count as meaning. It is always a mental event. I end my life without being aware that I had my head chopped off. Then my imagined post-mortem observation must be: the blade had no conscious meaning for my life. I did use it, however, so that its unconscious meaning had to be lived by me, however briefly. Whatever is, for me, means my wonderful being—expresses my mind and minds my expression. To particularize for the purpose of working up my self-view: my mind includes what I imagine. My mind includes my cloud. My mind includes my refuse. My mind includes my stars. My mind includes my drugs. My mind includes my jealousy, fear, and hate. My mind includes my submarine. My mind includes all of my wonderful universe. I may be careful of all of me. My mind includes all the ugly and repulsive aspects of my mind. My reader may fill in the blank to suit himself: My mind is ——.

The only possible trust *is* self-trust, and I am delighted whenever I live it confidently. Although my view of my individual life is such as to include all that I can be aware of living, I necessarily see myself as made up entirely of selfness, of individuality. Thus I see (my) you as a self, an individual comprising your whole world, but possibly now unable to appreciate your full wonderfulness and, hence, unable to care about it or care for it.

It is my refusal to acknowledge that my mind is living its any and every experience, which constitutes repression (self-dissociation into one fraction lived as self and another fraction lived as if not-self) and is the inception of deception. Yes, my refusal to acknowledge that my mind creates whatever I mean constitutes repression and is the beginning of mental disorder. Wherever my mind observes, wherever my mind smells, wherever my mind hears, wherever my mind tastes, and so on; if my mind refuses to acknowledge any of it as my mind experience, I do well to see how my mind is living itself. Thus I may see what my mind is doing to itself. It is in effect saying, "That is I," and

"That is not I," when in truth each is I. My all is I. This view gives me the answer to what and where my mind is. It is all about itself. The body-mind problem is seen to have foundation only in mind. The meaning "my body" is only a meaning. For me there is only my life. My promulgation of my body-mind problem may work to shut off this self-view; that is, it may have the meaning of repression.

"I quit again," cries my aroused reader, "and this time for good, if you keep hiding yourself behind these technical terms like 'repression.' I can see how you might forget where you put your glasses, but I don't see how you can forget where you put a piece of your own mind, and that, according to you, is 'repression.' "

Very well, when I forget where I put my glasses, I *am* only forgetting where I put a piece of my own mind, after all. Furthermore, you, yourself, alert reader, describe your writer as hiding, as hiding himself (from himself) behind his technical terms. In all truth, my repressed selfhood is its own repressing selfhood, quite as my resisting selfness is its own resisted selfness. Wherever the *universal* is not attributed to the *particular*, there repression is found.

To illustrate, if I do not attribute to *my* you (a particular of me) all of the properties of individuality which I claim for myself, then I thereby repress myself. It is the conscious self-observer who sees clearly that his enemy is solely and wholly his own creation, who recognizes sharply that a help to his enemy is a help to himself, and that a loss to his enemy is a loss to himself.

My everyone, or my everything, constitutes its own evidence, proof of being, and cannot be proved to exist through someone or something else. Hence, my lack of self-sight is represented in such a question as, "Can there be function without structure?" or "Can there be a 'mental' phenomenon unless 'we' posit a 'neurological' basis for it?" *Whatever of me is, is. Whatever of me is not, is not.* In this self-application each of these propositions of Parmenides still stands as the accurate guidepost for sanity.

"Halt in your onward rush of total disregard for anyone and everything *but* yourself, as being your tried and true way of self-helpfulness!" literally shouts my reader. "I am yet to be convinced that I cannot love a neighbor who is *not* my neighbor as well as I can love *my* neighbor. Show me how self-consciousness is anything except embarrassing, disconcerting, and bad-mannered. I have always associated it with weakness and demoralization, and as something to cure myself of. Now you ask me to turn completely around and go the opposite direction to my accustomed one!"

True, my self-consciousness is always extended against a first feeling of insecurity, of inconfidence. But my self-consciousness once developed is the very cure of my erstwhile feelings of inadequacy. There is nothing like tried self-consciousness for allaying every feeling of self-insufficiency, for delivering me from all of the signs that it (self-consciousness) is the one desideratum.

My awareness of my meaning, "full-measured self," embodies the truth that my mind is everything for me. To find (observe) all of my mind constitutes finding my everything, a process which in practice reduces to: I care for as much of my mind as I can recognize to be mine. My mind has many parts, some of which I have called by name in my book. If these are, in truth, as I observe them to be, the characteristics of my mind, then my selfness is comprehensive, all-inclusive and universal; and comprehensive self-awareness is a precious rarity. Mental material is my only material and its living is constituted of my living it. The fullest and clearest consciousness of my integration gives health; contrariwise, my living any part of myself without self-consciousness delivers that part of myself to the hazards of carelessness. In the latter predicament, the healthy warning signs, the helpful hand-maids of medicine and religion, commonly referred to disparagingly or with thinly veiled dislike as sickness, accident, sin, and evil, helpfully originate.

My individuality comprehends all of my human being. *It is not possible to observe, much less recognize, the whole of self in one view.* I observe myself only bit by bit. I live under the necessity of being divided from the conscious view of the all of my whole being. At any instant consciousness can reside only with that to which I am attending, but even that is most commonly an unacknowledged use of me, of my mind, of my selfness.

Predisposition of my mind to a *self-directed interpretation* of life appears to be a living of the nature of my universe. If I would preface every expression with the definition, "This is only about me," there could be no argument, speech would cease to be repressing, and my dictionary would begin to make truer sense.

Awareness of the truth that any and all points of view cannot contradict each other, or have anything to do with each other, is needed to settle all arguments well. In the first place, if it were possible for two people to be considering the same matter, there could be no argument.

The fact that they cannot possibly consider the same matter renders all argument futile. In the second place, no one person can make one out of two of his own points of view.

How frequently is heard my weak mind's lament, "I don't know what you mean," "What does it all mean?" or even, "What is the meaning of life?" How seldom is heard, "My everything is about me," "My all means I." The appreciation of my exclusive self-reliance grows as I exercise self-suppletive observations; e.g., all being is self-being, all expression is self-expression, all apparent otherness is self-otherness.

My Saint Augustine offers a description of the nature of God as a circle whose center is everywhere and circumference nowhere. I cannot in any way observe my existence other than as my own. My mind's creation of my concept, "myself and something else," is entirely and only a creation of my selfness. All plus another all is a contradiction in terms. The view that otherness applies to anything whatsoever but my own living must be seen kindly and tenderly so that it can be renounced. All recognized selfishness lends itself to renunciation, naught else can. The meaning "unselfishness" is in every instance the living of repressed selfishness.

By "renunciation" I mean nothing but living consciously as my human nature. By "renunciation," I mean essentially living on without relying upon repression (attempted self-disunion) for accomplishing it. "Renunciation" here means simply recognizing my living as my own but not being forced to be partial to it, either by over or under emphasis of it. Any life consciousness which I can see truly for its wonderfulness, I can renounce, that is, comfortably let go.

It does seem that it is necessary to live all of the values of religion as I extend my self-consciousness to include each one. I see no alternative to calling my life my own. I see benefit in such health imbuing living as adoration, reverence, and any and every other divine meaning.

I come to grief contending that my *imagining* what is external is not in every respect my own mental material. I am the origin of my universe. I am incapable of any living except what is innately original. My psychological work as a growing individual is that of living awareness as self-awareness. I am at my conception integrated, and all of my experiences are perfectly integrated in my being, and my mind strengthening work consists of consciously beholding this view. It is only right and solely supportable that I insist on my own world's unity. Thus, as a mentally mature person I have forced the growth of my insight that an effective way to look out for number one is to help make my world a better world to live itself in me. By the measure of self from a low estimate, to which it is commonly relegated, to what it truly is, namely, *all over,* I observe the facts of my life as from a higher ground. With this acknowledged identification with the *universal self,* what I really am, I observe that heedfulness and service to the needs of my others is nothing but preoccupation with self. Naturally I crown my good with brotherhood. Thus I grow to renounce giving immature reasons for helping myself, such as claiming to be able to help so-called "others." I see myself as staying on my original base. I am heart. I am my fellow man. Then, the sentence, "I am helping my fellow man by giving him a present," is seen as misreport or a lie. Then, the sentence, "I am helping myself by giving myself a present and getting a present from myself," is seen as accurate report or a truth.

The chief foible of my mind in trouble is its illusional self-expropriation, its hidden self-force, reminiscent of St. Matthew's parable of the buried talent. Therefore, the all important questioning for me is, "How much am I aware of living myself?" and "How much am I aware of being laid out in repudiated selfness which I use as my alias, others?" Idolatry represents an extreme form of self-deception. When I cannot call my soul my own, it is time for repentance, the beckoning signal for living at-*one*-ment. The illusional feeling of being at sixes and sevens in my own mind is dispelled by the appreciation that I am really at one, alone (all one). My Emerson had much of this idea in the following verses:

> There is no great and no small
> To the Soul that maketh all;
> And where it cometh, all things are;
> And it cometh everywhere.

The truth that an individual consists only of individuality cannot be stressed too much, for it says all that there is to say about the full-measured meaning of each and every human being. What place is there for blinding illusions of space or time in my Emerson's self-conscious living of his infinity and eternity?

> I am the owner of the sphere
> Of the seven stars and the solar year,
> Of Caesar's hand, and Plato's brain,
> Of Lord Christ's heart, and Shakspeare's strain.

XI. MY SELF-SCOPE

*All virtue and goodness tend to make men powerful in
the world; but they who aim at the power have not the
virtue.*

NEWMAN

THE DEVELOPING view of comprehensive human individuality attempts to treat all of selfhood as divine, god being
all; all being perfect and adorable, humanity being divine.
Healthy may be equated with holy; self with soul or spirit;
repression with atheism; apostasy, sacrilege, original sin,
with anarchy and damnation; sanative with sacred; universal with heavenly; self-sight or self-observation with
self-revelation; awareness of integration with salvation or
redemption; self-concern with prayer; conscious identification with blessing. Every one of my individual meanings
holds equally the one quality, that of being my own personal living. The sense of equality is the sense of sanity.

My Carlyle presented his concept of health in the following words: "It is a curious thing, which I remarked
long ago, and have often turned in my head, that of the old
word for 'holy' in the Teutonic languages, *heilig*, which

means 'healthy.' Thus *Heilbronn* means indifferently 'holy-well' or 'health-well.' We have in the Scotch, too, 'hale,' and its derivatives; and, I suppose, our English word 'whole' (with a 'w'), all of one piece, without any *hole* in it, is the same word. I find that you could not get any better definition of what 'holy' really is than 'healthy.' "

Observe the orientation of a consciously integrated man. He is aware of being his own world and he chooses to live this self-scope until he ends his life. He has to live whatever he creates. Whatever is for him good luck or bad luck, he has to live it as the best that he can live of his circumstances. He advises himself well to make the best of whatever he is. What he is, is. What he is not, is not. For him to grow in the direction of mental health means for him to live his necessity as himself. His mature religious orientation is to bow to the will of his god, which is his own, after all. The extension of his self-consciousness accomplishes the extension of his recognized will power. He sees his will of his god as his own will. His will and his divine will are one. He no longer separates himself from divine estimate. If he sees necessity as his own will, he is then theocratic in his life orientation. That level is not easy to achieve. In fact, he must work hard to achieve that reach. Thus, in his growing his ability to love his dislikes, he makes the best of his unpleasant living. Without self-consciousness his living force is loosely designated by such expressions of mental dissociation as "external necessity" and "internal compulsion."

My Descartes, the founder of modern philosophy, stated: "I think, therefore I am." This solipsism has been expressed innumerable times by every human seer in different words and in more or less epigrammatic manner as: my *philautia* of my ancient Greeks; my "egocentric predicament," or subjective monism, of my modern philosopher; my narcissism, autism, egoism of my modern psychiatrist; my rugged individualism of my economist; my inviolable soul of my clergyman; the I, me, or self of my man on the street. My Kant remarked: "This our world which is so real, with all its suns and milky ways, is nevertheless nothing but idea." And my Schopenhauer said: "This truth, which must be very serious and impressive if not awful to every one, is that a man can also say and must say, 'The world is my will.'" By "will" I can mean my mind's action, all of which may be subsumed under the much misunderstood term "imagination." I must *imagine* my perception, my sensation, quite as any other creation of mine. My Schopenhauer went on, "Now, since man is nature itself, and indeed nature at the highest grade of its self-consciousness, but nature is only the objectified will to live, the man who has comprehended and detained this point of view may well console himself, when contemplating his own death and that of his friends, by turning his eyes to the immortal life of nature, which he himself is." And on another occasion he wrote: "I say that he is his own work before all knowledge, and knowledge is merely added to enlighten it. Therefore he cannot resolve to be this or that, nor can he become other than he is; but he *is* once for all, and he knows in the course of experience *what* he is."

My physiologist Claude Bernard noted the organicity of the idea: "A cowardly assassin, a hero and a warrior each plunges a dagger into the breast of his fellow. What differentiates them, unless it be the ideas which guide their hands? A surgeon, a physiologist and Nero give themselves up alike to mutilation of living beings. What differentiates them also, if not ideas?" My Byron created this self-expression: "high mountains are a feeling."

In my existence, all parts of my mind are homogeneously alive. For instance, I use each one of my senses as a growth agency for developing my mind, for adding more parts to it. Its use is an integral process in my mental growth. While this sense is a means by which I live what I am, its usefulness, as my growing human being, is rarely seen clearly. I may believe, for example, that I see *something*, that *something* is cold, that *something* is warm, that *something* is touching me, that *something* is painful, that *something* "out there" is moving forward or backward outside of me, or externally around me, that I can taste *something* or that I can smell *something*, *other than myself*. I may persist in these delusions to the extent that it may never occur to me that my evidence of my sense is strictly self-grown self-evidence. Furthermore, the fierceness with which I argue that sense evidence is other than self-evidence, and that this otherness illusion has real existence apart from me, is the all-revealing clue that my will to uphold this delusion derives all of its force from my fierce will to live. A man who defends his external data as being external is really only defending the existence of his own life. Therefore, the illusion of externality, which can be only repressed internality, is stoutly defended as an unrecognized kind of self-preservation.

XII. I CREATE MY OPPOSITION

Today I was man and woman both, lover and mistress at once. I was riding through a forest on an autumn afternoon under the yellow leaves, and I was the horses, the leaves, the wind, the words that were spoken and the red sun that made them half close their eyelids drenched with love.

GUSTAVE FLAUBERT

IT IS NECESSARY to be exceedingly careful when I ask my fellow man to consider that his sense experience is totally his growing of self-experience—evidence of the human being which he is living. For instance, when I ask my fellow man to consider that he cannot see anybody or anything else, only himself, and that this view is to be taken literally and not in any figurative sense, *that* may be a trying assignment for him, as it often is for me. It is much easier for me to read Descartes, Schopenhauer, Bernard or Byron, each at his self-conscious best, sense the flavor of the saying, and ignore these observations as being my important living. So confused (self-distracted) am I, on occasions, about this truth of my own inviolable individuality, that I am tempted to disregard its health significance.

97

Every living of self-consciousness is health recoupment. The health habit of mind is the habit of self-consciousness, a vital devotion distinguishing presence of mind from absent-mindedness.

Certain expressions which I use for describing my persevering in conscious self-growth are of interest: "coming to life again," "the great awakening," "giving up death in life," "coming out of a trance," "I feel different, steadier," "I'm turning over a new leaf," "I get very lonesome, but better," "I'm showing more life," "I see how mixed up I am and I don't like it," "It's hard to take, but there it is," "I'm seeing that the outer man is really the inner man, myself," "This work makes me think of a quotation from Saint Bernard, 'We must retire inward, if we would ascend upward,'" "Self-consciousness is truly fine, but I don't have the time to devote to it," "I have to work too hard at growing more self-unconsciousness," "I can see now that there is no possibility of a right view of what I call 'anything else' before I have a right view of my own being," "I used to take one look at all the things I didn't like and I'd say to myself, 'I'd rather be nuts but happy, than miserably sane'; I never admitted before that living well required any seeing to it," "I always thought pain was to be relieved by analgesics. You ask me to sharpen my consciousness where it hurts."

When I am living, hence working, at the level of self-rejection, my self-repudiation may be expressed in one of these ways: "It's too deep for me," "If that's so, why don't other educators teach that," "When I am self-conscious, I am disconcerted. That's enough evidence for me that it doesn't work well," "Where ignorance is bliss, it's folly to be wise," "You have one philosophy of mind, and I have another," "I want to be a scientist, not a philosopher," "I don't like this study," "If you don't count in my life, what are you doing here; why are you teaching?" "It takes less exertion for me to study than it does for me to study myself, and I am just about exhausted at the end of each day as it is," "You make too much out of what you claim is the necessity to take care of yourself in order to live well," "Why can't you talk the way other people talk," "You take words and thrust them out of their normal connotation and use them to suit yourself," "Everybody knows that selfishness is reprehensible, but you call it adorable," "I don't want to be like other people and you say I have to be my other people. I say *no* to that," "You say I sleep my other people, but I say you dream that you are your own other people," "You ask me to create a nervous breakdown. I say let sleeping dogs lie," "You say such sleeping dogs as rejected human elements get expressed physiologically in organ dysfunction. I say that physiologists would have found that out long ago if it were true," "Your teachings upset me, and health education should set me up," "You say you can be cheerful about feeling sad. I call that crazy talk," "You seem friendly, but I just can't like you the way you are," "Self-consciousness makes me scatterbrained, but I can concentrate my mind on external data."

My beginning student soon asks: "How can you enjoy your work if you don't feel that you are helping your fellow man? How do you satisfy yourself in your teaching and therapy, if you don't feel that you're instructing the ignorant and curing the sick?" My treatment of this puzzlement is first of all to observe that it is wonderful questioning, then to ask the consideration: "May I not feel happy if I enjoy the view of my student *growing his self-knowledge,* and of my patient *healing himself,* recovering his own health? Is not my satisfaction complete in my seeing my fellow man using and prizing his true power sources? Would I not have to feel somewhat as a medical kidnapper if I were to try vainly to usurp my patient's right to find his helpfulness where it truly is for him, within himself?"

Next my student asks: "But how is education ever possible if you can't tell another anything and can't even learn from example?" Again, only after honoring the query, after "respecting the burden," I continue: "Does not my realization that *my* teaching is entirely a matter of my own living allow me to observe that I have grown, not given or received, my lesson? Is not my awareness that I grow my own sensations, perceptions, and viewpoints, a benefit over and above any illusion that I have unloaded them on someone else or had someone else unload them on me? Is it not immediately my own, that which I create by my living? Must I deceive myself that I can expropriate or appropriate it *unnaturally?* Perhaps my appreciation of individuality may seem extreme, *but is not the extreme of one still one?*"

As I progress in cultivating the habit of self-observation, I notice that I increase exercises of earnestness, seriousness, deep sincerity, careful concern, and similar evidence of proper self-regard; conversely, I observe myself renouncing the exercise of such feelings as carelessness, flippancy, recklessness, indolence, suspicion, gloom, stagefright, envy, and similar evidences of disrespect. In other words, *in my growth of this habit of self-consciousness I find my con-*

sideration for my others becoming greater rather than less.
Only self-interest can quicken my considerateness, and
every one of my human beings in my life presents idio-
syncrasies requiring tender consideration.

XIII. I OBSERVE MYSELF
PIECEMEAL

Every materialist will be an idealist; but an idealist can never go backward to be a materialist.

The idealist, in speaking of events, sees them as spirits. He does not deny the sensuous fact: by no means; but he will not see that alone. He does not deny the presence of this table, this chair, and the walls of this room, but he looks at these things as the reverse side of the tapestry, and the other end, each being a sequel or completion of a spiritual fact which merely concerns him. This manner of looking at things transfers every object in nature from an independent and anomalous position without there into the consciousness. Even the materialist Condillac, perhaps the most logical expounder of materialism, was constrained to say: "Though we should soar into the heavens, though we should sink into the abyss, we never go out of ourselves; it is always our own thought that we perceive." What more could an idealist say?

EMERSON

IF EACH one must live his own world, how then can anyone acquire any conviction at all that there is existence besides his own? *This question poses a true phantom problem.*

My external-world view is just as much a use of my imagination as is any other view that I grow. The attribute "externality" is one which is best seen clearly from start to finish as nothing but the property of repressed selfness. To exalt self-repudiation over self-consciousness as a way of living is to hold that reasoning, including full-blown delusion, is superior to esteemed sensible individuality as a health principle.

No moment of my living allows for total self-awareness, total self- appreciation, total self-esteem, total self-meaning. However, I can imagine that I am able to have such a view. I can imagine my feeling every element of my being, but the actual living of my self-appreciation is a piecework operation. I overwhelm myself when I attempt to live myself consciously *in toto*. I stun my capacity for concentrated attention when I attempt to sense my totality.

This single insight that only a part of me can live consciously one self-scene at a time is of the greatest helpfulness. It is helpful in dispelling my illusion that when I say, "Yes" to any of my living or "No" to any of my living, that all of me is thereby saying, "Yes" or "No." If I indulge my illusion that my "Yes" already means that *all of me* is favorably disposed to a proposition, I thereby spare myself the feeling of necessity to affirm the matter further, but also I thereby exclude myself from any such opportunity. It is of the greater health benefit for me to see clearly that any and every moment of my conscious living is momentary surface production.

Everyone of my world observes the ease with which he can deceive himself about the degree to which he has learned his lesson. When I am conscious that I do not like some, or any, of my living, it is obvious that all of me is not thereby bent upon rejection, for *I am my all* and therefore must cherish as my life all of my living which I reject. However, by indulging my illusion that all of me is solidly enforced against some of my living, I can escape the realization that I am actually hurting myself in the process. Certainly it is helpful for me to be able to see that I live my own rejected living, that is, that I am capable of living myself unkindly (and shall certainly do so to the extent that I live myself unconsciously).

My fall-of-man occurs when I start to use my senses without accepting my sensory living as evidence of my self-growth only. This form of self-rejection, of my disowning my fruit of my own tree of knowledge, represents my fall as man. When I use my signification not-I, without realizing that such is a self-use entirely, then I immediately set up a self-deception which implies that I am able to lose my mind. I do not pretend to lose all of it. No matter how much I use my not-I illusion, there always remains a nucleus felt as I. With this (however restricted) nucleus I may, and must, hold the delusion that I am using *all* of my right mind. The scientific fact is that I am my own *all,* and that for me to delude myself that I can live anything beside myself is an evident instance of inaccuracy. I cannot accurately express all, plus (or minus) anything. If anything can be added to it, it was not *all* to begin with; if anything can be subtracted from it, it was not *all* to begin with.

The following description spells out this plight of my fall-of-man: I have grown an environment in myself in which I can find security through considering that I am insignificant. By claiming to be a nobody I can at least live my necessity to be a somebody. I live feelings of approval by disowning vast tracts of my human being. I attain a developmental level indicating that I feel like a somebody, but the route is *via* calling myself a nobody. I feel very much like a human being by complying with my self-restricting forces, or elements, for instance, with each of my intolerant parent figures (individuations of my individuality). But so much of myself is repudiated (disclaimed) by my *accepted me* that, as far as my own acknowledgment of myself is concerned, I am a fraction of a man. Thus I spend my life in name calling, this is "good" but that is "bad," this is "right" but that is "wrong," this is "I" but that is "not-I," this is "scientific" but that is "unscientific," this is "sacred" but that is "profane," this is "humane" but that is "unhumane." I am doing my best to live myself as a goner.

Unless I realize that every action of mine has to do with me, *and me only*, I cannot recognize that my instinct to live is one for all of my self-preservation, and hence, one for the care of all of my universe. *I* am not ill; *I* probably cannot be all ill and live. However, some of my conduct may be helpfully out of order and my other conduct struggling more on that account. Such ordeals, in which I find the going tough, I may designate as "my illness." My illness may express itself in a part of my physiology. I may even suffer liver trouble, heart trouble, or family trouble without in any way realizing such illness as a healthy sign that I am not taking the trouble to keep my self-consciousness in line with my self-growth. My physiology thereby has not gone to pieces, in any undesirable sense. Every physiological sign of my troubled living is of indispensable helpfulness for my regaining my equilibrium as a health-fully living individual. That means, in its effort to signalize my mental dissociation, one of my organ systems functions to advance itself at the cost of another, and thus I must live physiological compensations and decompensations.

How can I see my illness as helpful, as life affirming? Surely it is a precious sign to me of the way in which I am living myself. I cannot well go against my best interests without having the signs of such waywardness appear. I can ignore the meaning of every such sign as meaning off the track of appropriate self-appreciation, if I have not developed the skill to decipher it.

To what extent is my own language of ill health entirely a foreign language to me and resisted as such? Once I see the meaning of my health sign and decide to pay profitable attention to it, I devote myself to concerning myself about elements of my selfhood which I have habitually ignored. This is my devotion to my mending my way of life. I begin to center myself consciously in my living. I see my mind as *all in its own place*. I renounce my habit of disowning myself in my addiction to subordinating my real self-view of space, or time, or motion, to an illusional self-view of space, or time, or motion. I no longer practice my illusion of getting out of bed, or going from one place to another, but enjoy the real sense of selfhood in *growing* every such movement and place. I renounce name calling: this is "good" that is "bad," this is "I" but that is "not-I," this is "scientific" but that is "unscientific," this is "sacred" but that is "profane."

"It seems to me, according to your account," interjects my reader, "that in order to understand myself now, all I have to do is find out how I grew to understand myself in the first place. Was I aware that I was *all I* to begin with? Did I start my life on the right track of self-, and only self-, conscious growth?

The scientific fact is that I gave birth to myself as a complete individual, and, as such, I had no other possible way of living myself. As I developed myself I used a way of avoiding painful living by ignoring it as much as possible. Quite an anaesthetic, this ignoration! An excellent device for my ignoring my painful living was to call it "not-mine." By identifying my likable living as my own but classifying my dislikes as not mine, I made my unpleasant living only my unconscious (ignored) living. Thus I deliver out of my conscious living of it, into my unconscious living of it, as much of my unpleasant living as I can. Now right here is where I have to cut off my nose to spite my face, for what I make my unconscious living I thereby make my involuntary living. True, I succeed in forgetting my unpleasant experience and, by not having it conscious, do not have it accessible for (what would be painful) conscious use. Thus I succeed in feeling irresponsible for any personal need to hurt myself or to feel hurt. I can always account to myself for any distress or unpleasantness by considering it of foreign origin. On the other hand, all of my unconscious living being involuntary living, the more it accrues the less available conscious will power (stamina, morale, purposiveness, workability, etc., based upon volition) I have, and the more available unconscious will power (habit, obstinacy, defiance, resistance, impulsiveness, attacks, spells, etc., based upon involuntary force) I have. Obviously, the conscious disposition of my living, so that my conscious living accrues, contributes in every way to my appreciation of my self-power and the happy sense of self-esteem corresponding with this full-measured self-evaluation. My misunderstanding of myself is traceable in its entirety to my not making myself persistently a potentially conscious self and to my persistently maintaining my amnesia for whatever unconscious self-living I can, by means of that missing link, not-I.

XIV. DISCOVERING UNITS
OF MYSELF

They drew a circle to shut him out—
Heretic, rebel, a thing to flout.
But Love and I had the wit to win:
We drew a circle that took him in!

EDWIN MARKHAM

IN CHART III, I refer to human living and to self-discovery and draw it without plotting a curve on it. I see clearly the health necessity for growing myself consciously, particularly throughout any part of my life which develops in a surprising kind of rapidity. However, I am unable to plot my curve in view of certain facts. To mention certain prominent complication factors, first of all I am not aware of my age when my first glimmering of self-consciousness is lived. Furthermore my self-consciousness has always been lived as a momentary surface insight without further self-depth or duration. Also, every living of my self-consciousness has constituted its own unique quality and quantity of self-consciousness.

Self-discovery, first of all, is the only possibility of *dis-*

covery. Consciousness of it as being the only possibility introduces the true economy of living. Discovery, defined, must mean self-growth associated with the feeling that it is oneself which is grown and which is doing all the growing.

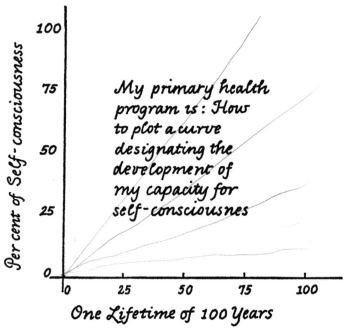

CHART III. *The Development of My Capacity for Self-consciousness*

As before noted, I may grow myself without this kind of self-appreciation *only at the cost of my diminishing estimate of the greatness of my being.* By recognizing that my growth is my only self-possession, I force myself to esteem the one and only truth for me: my self-development is my self-fulfillment, self-realization, self-working harmoniously, self-creating my own world, self-augmenting with every experience of my homogeneous creaturehood.

I cannot apply myself, work myself well, except to the extent that I recognize this employment as my living of *me*. Conscious self-application begets conscious self-application and thus furthers my insight upon my power as a worker. Do I work well? is the same question as, Does my life run smoothly? I find that every development of my function of my capacity for applying myself consciously, for working well, is in every instance sensed as an access of happiness. To make an epigram of it: He who works himself consciously the most is the happiest. He who works himself consciously the least is the unhappiest. My ability to work myself consciously has a manifestation in the ability of the body part of my mind (my physiology) to function harmoniously.

Discovery is thus observable as nothing but self-growth. Making discovery conscious is nothing but making self-growth conscious. A clear disadvantage in growing myself, discovering myself, without observing it as mine, is the lack of a proper self-estimate, and every hazard of shackled selfness which such unacknowledged living entails. Particularly, my scientific imagination suffers from this mental road blocking. Every kind of mental disorder has as its one and only indispensable disordering force: restriction of self-observation.

Self-proof is fool proof. Self-certainty is true certainty. As a scientist, I am avowedly interested in the facts of immediate experience. My living, only, provides me with these facts. The fact of myself furnishes the essence of anything and everything factual in my scientific work. My science of self underlies all of my science. The fiction of not-self is seen most truthfully as nothing but another fact of self. Where I must say, "It is not I," I must forego accuracy.

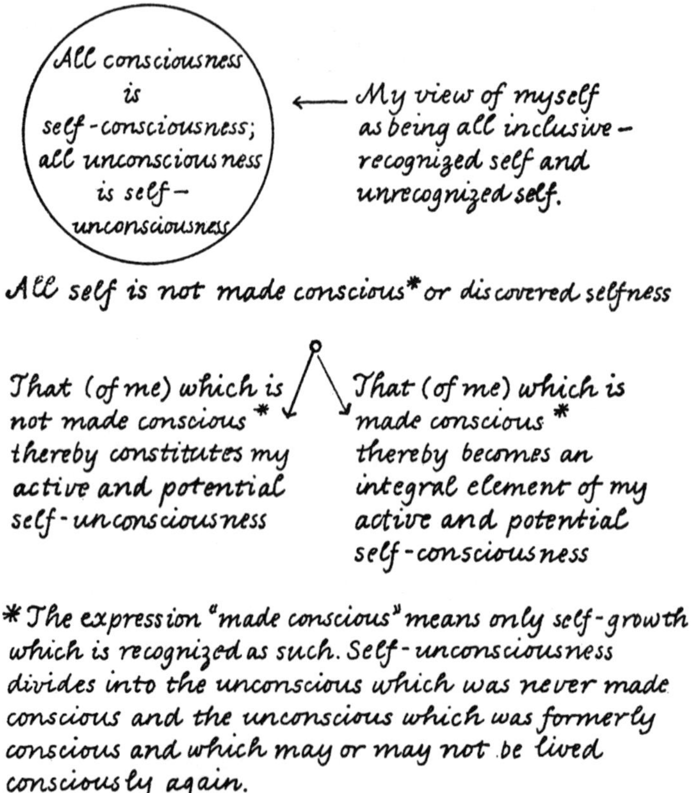

All consciousness is self-consciousness; all unconsciousness is self-unconsciousness

← My view of myself as being all inclusive – recognized self and unrecognized self.

All self is not made conscious* or discovered selfness

That (of me) which is not made conscious* thereby constitutes my active and potential self-unconsciousness

That (of me) which is made conscious* thereby becomes an integral element of my active and potential self-consciousness

* The expression "made conscious" means only self-growth which is recognized as such. Self-unconsciousness divides into the unconscious which was never made conscious and the unconscious which was formerly conscious and which may or may not be lived consciously again.

CHART IV. *My Human Individuality with Reference to its Conscious and Unconscious Vitality*

Discovering Units of Myself

Without question, every problem of my world is necessarily my problem. Without question, my world has many a problem of which I am unconscious. However, here again, my unconsciousness of any problem of mine cannot make it no problem of mine. My awareness of any problem of my world is necessary for my seeing it as my own; however, my unawareness of any problem of my world, does not cancel its meaning as being my own.

XV. MY WORD LIFE

*The better things are understood the more are they
found beautiful and comfortable to the desires which a
wise man might form.*

VON LEIBNITZ

IN MY Dryden's apt phrase, "Sense flows in fit words." My
every word is a living element of me. My experimental activity, science, depends upon a kind of sober acquiescence
with what I am living and observing as being my living.
What is of me *is,* and what is not of me *is not.* There is a
need for a word descriptive of every way in which I live my
mind, descriptive of every kind of my mental activity. The
word "dream" might be used were it not for the fact that it
already carries the false connotation of being unreal. What
is, is real. "Unreal" is another word for negation of reality.
The word "cerebrate" carries with it the false connotation
that it is a non-mental process. Whatever meaning *is,* is
mental. The word "mentate" carries with it little or no
familiarity. What meaning it has tends to imply restricted
living. Perhaps the truest word for describing any and
every kind of mental activity is the term "living" itself.
In order that a wonderful word may thereby be rescued

from varying degrees of repression as a mental activity, I choose that very one to describe any and all mental activity, the word "imagine." To say that I have no imagination is to describe myself as suffering *rigor mortis*. To say that I have a lively imagination is to describe myself as man alive. To the extent that I am able to see that my external world in every single respect is an imagined one is essential for me to be able to call my soul my own. With this view my science is consciously humanized. Without it I live as if I can dehumanize my science.

In living (growing) my activity called "perceiving," it helps to be consciously mindful that I am *imagining*. How then am I able to tell whether I am actually perceiving, or actually hallucinating, if each is all imagination? My imagining my *perception* which I designate as my mental object, involves a kind of living distinct from my imagining my mental object *without employing my sensory organ for* accomplishing it. How am I aware of the difference? In the same way that I am aware of any and every difference, really—simply by virtue of the fact that I live each one in a way peculiar to it alone.

My method of experimental science is essentially empirical, involving the growing of my (self-) observations in the form of my sensations and my perceptions. I examine and study these new developments as constant increments of self-growth, as progressive augmenting of my conscious self-totality. Perception issues from the actual growing of sensory experience. My interpretation of induction is that it consists of the systematic growth and ordering of perceptions.

The trouble with a definition is that it may, and usually

does, imply that one thing can have something to do with another, an obvious impossibility. The work recorded in this volume is for the express purpose of pointing up the health value of *practiced* self-consciousness. Each word is intended as an end in this direction in the sense that its *indispensable* definition is its meaning as a word of, about, and for myself. However, within this all important frame of reference (that is, every term's meaning is an element of my living), the following terms are used in the sense described after them.

Sensation: is all and only about mental life produced entirely through the living of an organ of sense.

Perception: is all and only about direct living recognition that the life produced by a sense organ has existence, is a mental object.

Conception: is all and only about the living (conceiving) of an idea, notion, or understanding.

Induction: is all and only about the living of an exposition of observational (self-) evidence supplied by a sequence, or class, of perceptions. Induction is an instance of the arrival of the particular at the general (universal).

Deduction: is all and only about the living of an exposition of a sequence, or class, of perceptions thereby attributing the meaning of a general conception to the several perceptions. Deduction is an instance of the arrival of the general (universal) at the particular.

Feeling or Emotion: is all about itself, the living of mental elements accounting for the varying degrees of pleasure and pain.

Apperceiving: is all and only about the exciting (activation) of already grown perceptions, thus directing attention to, and thereby electing the growth of, sensations and perceptions satisfying to those already grown.

Consciousness: is all and only about a living of wakefulness, awareness enabling appreciation of being alive.

Experimental Science: is all and only about the investigation of my mental life by experiment (prearranged method).

Selfness: is all and only about individuality, existence, unique identity, one-ness, entity, homogeneous unity, mind, soul, all.

Imagination: is all and only about mental activity of every kind (in this work). What is not imagined is meaningless, and *meaninglessness* is a synonym for nothing.

Reality: is all about whatever is; whatever is, is real. An illusion is a real illusion, an error is a real error, a negation is a real negation.

Adding sensation to my organ's living may be considered as analogous to adding feeling to my mind's somatic activity, or adding perception to my mental object's existence, or adding consciousness to my view of creaturehood *in toto.* My growth of sensation, perception, or consciousness is the development of my mind. The utility of my mental work, as in study, is not so much the growth of self-knowledge in the form of dogmatic truths, or of insights, as it is the development of greater capacity for *mind working,* itself, and the life satisfaction derivable from this evolving maturation of my mind. *That* I live me in my marvelous variety is the source of my health giving self-esteem.

I may look at my radiator with the use of my eye and not be able to say what the radiator-ness of the sensation is at all, if I do not enliven (imagine) my particular apperception: what radiator means. To employ apperception is to use deduction, rather than induction, and entails no further *growth* of peripheral organs of sensation. As I use my sensory apparatus for living a view (of myself) which I designate "radiator," I may make up my mind (imagine) that it is of cardboard, in view of the fact that my apperceptions introduce that deduction. With further directed living of my sensory apparatus, I might enable myself to decide that my radiator is made of plywood. I start to make further inductions from there, and still upon closer inspection of the new grown sensation, decide (imagine) that my radiator is made of iron. Next I realize that I am on my stage in my theatre, and I use my inductive imagination again, and sense further by sight, hearing, and touch of my radiator. Finally I employ more apperception, and deduce that my radiator is made of plastic, is a convenient prop on my stage. Imagination is the working of my mind, applying to apperceptions as well as to perceptions and sensations. Sensory experience is always a new self-growth involving immediate living of my sensory apparatus. Once grown, my sensation is lived as a perception, and as a perception thereafter it accrues to augment my system of apperceptions.

An ever present limitation of reasoning is the extent to which it utilizes apperceptive material. My reasoning lends itself every bit as much to the construction of a paranoiac system as of a philosophical rationale. All of my reality is psychic reality. As my Freud has pointed out, my reality testing does not consist simply of the growth of a sensation or perception. Rather it consists of my finding a familiarity for what I am perceiving with what I had formerly perceived. Reality testing is illusional, if the reality meaning is not a self-felt one. My reality testing actually involves my growing a perception, and then growing a realization (consciousness) of its being mine. *My certainty feeling associated with my making it conscious at will is my (psychic) reality testing.*

My reader now takes over: "Will you please deign to make your reader a psychic reality of yours? Are you aware of the degree to which you are having him test his own sense of what is real? If you sense your identity in your reader, how can you throw your weight around, realizing that your reader, in all probability, has not worked and worded his mind precisely as you have worked and worded yours?"

I cannot make any claim whatsoever upon the understanding or tolerance of my reader—only he can do that. Furthermore, I cannot recommend *Living Consciously: The Science of Self* to my reader as being a helpful way of life for him—only he can do that. I do all that I can do in describing how I have learned how to help myself, by trying to make an accurate language for studying the living of myself.

XVI. JUMPING THE TRACK OF SELF-CONSCIOUSNESS

It is not the mere cry of moralists, and the flourish of rhetoricians; but it is noble *to seek truth, and it is* beautiful *to find it. It is the ancient feeling of the human heart —that knowledge is better than riches; and it is deeply and* sacredly true!

SYDNEY SMITH

IF I HAD a systematic vocabulary for it, I might describe myself as a soul or spirit or universe or divine impetus. From the standpoint of order and accuracy it is necessary that my developing human being accompany its growth with its appreciation that it is its own growing. This is a rare revelation. I tend to grow myself without the realization that *that* is all that can be. I am all of my own mind, no more and no less. My very first growth of what I call "not-self," is the product of my mind's capacity to say "No" in such a way that I affirm the contradiction: What is, *is* not. The mental function of negation serves to spare my baby mind otherwise overwhelming tensions. My first traumatic mental experience is paradigmatic of all to follow, consisting essentially of the mental imposture: It is not I. My baby resort to negation may be pictured somewhat as follows: I have a wish which leads me to seek for direct gratification at the same time that I grow a perception, as a powerful counterforce, a perception which I later call "mother" or "father." My drive toward gratification and my inhibiting pressure are felt by me as painful tension which I later call "anxiety." In this mental circumstance I find myself seeking gratification in two exclusive ways. *My counterforce which I develop is every bit as much I as is my primitive instinctive need.* As this action system of counterforces augments in my individuality, I find myself living my human being in multitudinous ways. Out of all that I live I gradually consolidate some appreciation of myself as a unity. It appears evident that I am never able actually to include all of myself in any deliberate measure of myself.

"Why not?" questions my reader. "Why can't I simply realize that I am my own all-that-is, all-that-was, and all-that-ever-will-be? It seems to me, if I can imagine as true much of what I have just been reading, I should have no trouble in letting my imagination soar a little higher. According to you, I use up my precious imagination chiefly by *imagining* that *my* external world is *not mine*. Maybe so, maybe so. Maybe not so, too. I have a large acquaintance with imagination running wild, and I acknowledge a proper fear of it. Suppose I'd imagine you to be *my* you—perish the thought!"

Yes, it is possible, as I have my you bring out, for me to imagine anything at all, including my imagining that I can imagine seeing all of myself all at once. However, it is a self-evident fact that every one of my self-views is all and only about itself and therefore does not, and cannot, subsume all of the rest of my self-views! Yes, I do find my fellow man using up his precious imagination in order to imagine that his own external world is corpse cold as far as his living of any of it is concerned.

Two forces facilitate negation: the repelling force of the exclusiveness of my accepted self and the drawing power of my habitually rejected self. In growing myself as a child I may live my mother, father, sibling, and my everyone else in the form of disclaimed selfness. I am not really conscious that all of this living of otherness is entirely my own. I cannot but speculate on the meaning of this constitutional deception as a health problem. As I grow a certain set of meanings in my life which I denominate "fellow man," which seems to me to stand for great power, it is most easy for me to grow the *illusion* that my he is not a part of me, that my every sensation or every perception is not a self out-growth of my internality, but is an ingrowth of (not my) externality. And such self-deception occurs whenever, as a parent, I live any meaning of my child without recognizing it as my own. This self-repudiation is less apt to be true to the extent that, as a parent, I represent an equalitarian, libertarian, solitarian kind of living. I would be most unusually fortunate to grow as the latter kind of parent, whose child's parental meaning would be entirely compatible with the rest of his child's growing of self-sight. I can gladly imagine the health meaning of my nicely coordinating physiology associated with my comprehensive self-sight.

XVII. MY SCIENTIFIC I

In so far as it places all phenomena on the same emotional level, the scientific point of view may be called the God's-eye view.

J. B. S. HALDANE

I OBSERVE my godliness when I see that I can do no wrong. The grandeur of this ethical statement is unsurpassed. When I develop the insight that whatever is is right, that everything must be in its necessities just, I thereby behold *the soul stirring truth that I never did anything wrong in my life* and that it is impossible for me ever to do anything wrong. With this observation I can renounce my enormous investment of my valuable guilt feelings in blame and reproach and utilize the energy thus made available for profitable investment in becoming responsible for my selfhood. My mind's capacity to designate one part of itself as "good" and another part of itself as "bad" is a highly valuable kind of primitive reflex which is most useful for first screening of varying degrees of helpful experience. All of me has its place, even the concept of right and wrong. It is desirable to be able to react to injury reflexly with pain; I do not, therefore, consider my life to be dominated by pain. Why therefore have it dominated by the feeling of wrong (depression and accusation)?

I can make trouble for myself in my area called (self-ignorantly) "relationships," by claiming blindly that what is need not be. There is nothing wrong about any mental material, even about self-disesteem, even about its not being seen as my own wonderful mental material. There is only one kind of name calling which is sane, namely, calling (whatever) my own name. Why is criticism never scientific either in letter or spirit? In both it carries the implication of prejudice against what is. There is no contending against facts, no use arguing against whatever is, as Newton observed.

My organized, but self-unconscious, mind blindly plays some kind of system for its plan of operation. My gears go through their cycle. In contrast, when my self-conscious mind controls, I can observe what is advantageous and disadvantageous and can feel my way. My only true common sense is my I feeling, sensed as being common to my whole person. The I, or me, feeling clears my mind for the appropriate operation of my self-interest principle, so that my sentiment of self-preservation can act for self-help (and against self-hurt) with its natural force. *The insensibility of my unobserved selfness is my greatest liability.* By concentrating my attention upon any one mental part, most easily a word, I may observe that it soon begins to make no sense. Thus I am warned by my own human being that I do well to keep my attention mobile, that there is more to me than any one part, and that any portion of my mental material derives its healthiest meaning in terms of the full flowing vigor of all of my psychic content.

My most wholesome view of apparent loss is to chalk it up to experience, let bygones immediately be bygones, and proceed in a kind, life affirming way of living.

My basic principle of psychology is *life, living*. I live the only life it is possible to live. It is for the purpose of being enjoyed. I become ill by losing track of the main issue of enjoying my life by realizing that it is. There is no aspect or phase of my life which is not to be regarded as enjoyable—whether birth, sickness, or death. Joy of living is health giving recognition of living.

I start myself enjoying life in any way in which I can please myself. Then as I grow, I work out ways of enjoying my life which involve more and more of myself. But I never lose track of the main idea that I am alive for the purpose of enjoying myself. There is no truer way of life. Getting the most enjoyment out of my life involves finding out the most of myself. The joy of living is my only unfailing incentive to live myself fully, which fullness in turn insures living myself well, including morally. Through impersonal (enforced) morals I cannot find a way to joyful living, try and deceive myself as I may and frequently do. True to life living kindles health. What is my goal in life? I can only answer to live. If I wish to elaborate on this idea, it is impossible, except to say "to live fully," by which I mean basically, "do all of my own living consciously and want more of it." There is no substitute for living. There is no substitute for being. Whatever is, extremely is; whatever is not, extremely is not.

Self-interest is the only possible basis for developing healthy manhood or womanhood. As infant and child I prove myself proficient in looking out for my narrowly conceived self. Then I succeed to increments of self-awareness until I am able to oversee my broadly conceived self. The signification of self is ever reverent. *To have the highest moral worth an action must be motivated by acknowledged self-interest.* Any other so-called moral principles cannot possibly be true to life, hence must fail. If I ask myself, "How do I know?" the idea presents itself: The same way I know anything at all; namely, I observe it, and every self-observation is known by its works.

When I sense, perceive, and observe that I am only treating myself well in having my (imagined) neighbor treat himself well, I have the only trustworthy moral safeguard. Self-love is the only valid universal law of life which admits of no equivalent.

When I look at myself with the insight that I am looking at myself, and then realize that my self-scenery is the only place which I can possibly see, I sense the great value of an attitude of self-devotion. It is what I have before called "the divine look," one constituting the keenest, brightest kind of attention. Whenever I find myself not using my divine look, I thereby create for myself the problem of evil, which latter is a blessed sign that I am attempting to live well by dispensing with the healing and strengthening value of seeing my all from the clearest point of view. When I attempt to dissociate my divine look, by considering it as something that is above or beyond or attempt to imprison it in any way, this constitutes my most dangerous form of dissociation. This dissociation is best designated kindly for what it is—my atheistic viewpoint.

If I set my heart on honesty I must attribute divinity to

my criminality as to all else. I have been, and am always, doing all that is possible. My criminal's contracted concept of selfhood accounts for his shortsighted self-helpfulness. When my imagined help seeker voices his difficult thoughts and feelings (including all action), he is seeking to help himself to find their wholesome enjoyable use. If I am unable to mind my imagined fellow man's trouble as my own useful mental material, and instead resort to ignoring it as being my own, I reduce myself to the immature life status of "fighting the devil with his own weapons."

To be alive is to be experiencing self. That is all possible. According to this viewpoint, it is rare for one of my imagined people to live himself fully. I can live more fully, but only if I can learn to tolerate more of myself. I can extend my self-tolerance only by acknowledging more necessities in my ever growing self. To live fully is to support "the weight of centuries" good-naturedly instead of only mean spiritedly, "to take arms against a sea of troubles" well disposedly instead of only "sicklied o'er with the pale cast of thought." To live fully is to learn from experience that my instinctive repudiation of truth, necessity, is sufficient explanation of all of my guilt. To live fully is to learn from experience that failure, compliance, obedience are also life savers. I can only be truly virtuous when I learn from experience to make a virtue of necessity. "God's will be done," says the religious one of everything that is, as the indispensable beginning for happier living.

What is the alternative to making the best of it? Burns remarked: "We become men, not after we have been dissipated, and disappointed in the chase of false pleasure; but after we have ascertained, in any way, what impassable barriers hem us in through this life; how mad it is to hope for contentment to our infinite soul from the gifts of this extremely finite world; that a man must be sufficient for himself; and that for suffering and enduring there is no remedy but striving and doing. Manhood begins when we have in any way made truce with Necessity; begins even when we have surrendered to Necessity, as the most part only do; but begins joyfully and hopefully only when we have reconciled ourselves to Necessity; and thus, in reality, triumphed over it, and felt that in Necessity we are free."

Why, for example, do I have the tremendous feeling of power driving me on? I can feel that I have no place to turn to, no place to go. In that situation I invariably have not acquired the insight that I am the only place that there is. It helps me to ask myself what I amount to, what I add up to, and to find out that what I have been calling myself has too seldom been my rightful name. I notice that I have repudiated large tracts of myself, that I have disregarded that feeling of self which is tremendous and invigorating.

I can worship myself and adore myself in my real life, instead of in a phantom elsewhere. That is the big idea of my living. And yet I may live to an advanced age and find that I have taken all this which is myself and I have put it some place in myself which I call: "the church," "friend," "child," "science," "job," "stock market," "bonds," "car," "flowers," "boat," "foreign lands." And soon I have turned away from all of this of myself, as if I could put something wonderful outside of me to behold it as separate from me. I have deprived myself of the source of help which comes from my truthfulness, humility, sincerity, piety, from the perfectly natural thoughts and feelings of my human being.

An effort on the part of one great division of my humanity (which is I also) to be helpful is my religious one. As church man I treat what I call disease of my soul, or I may not even call it disease of the soul. In my religion I work with my personal means. I work on the level of personal meaning—with what I call spirituality. Perhaps the word "spiritual" can also connote "externality," but insight can dispel that illusion too. This view needs presentation in a most candid way to be considered for its great value in promoting healthful self-esteem. I can arouse my resistance to my comment that my fellow man, who is helping himself with divinity, is entirely self-contained. As a thoroughly self-conscious person, I see myself working on all of me there is to work on, with all there is to work with, in the interest of the life of my developing human being. But it is easy for me, from force of habit of self-disregard, to take the position, "This 'easy' street is one way for me to have my feeling of being O.K. It means I do not know how sick I am, and I am no different from any of my other billions of people in my world who have arrived at this compromise within themselves, of calling themselves well because they ignore how sick they are." That is the way my demagog has ever lived, dealt with his illness by denying its existence. A human life is a strenuous one and is best lived with that insight. I must work well or ill.

The doctrine of self-insight holds the greatest possible sanative power and enables the development of the best level of human being. It offers greatest healthfulness in mental living. It prepares all advances in wellness and goodness, endowing such honored expressions as the following with their greatest sense:

Physician heal thyself

The kingdom of God is within you

Love thine enemy

I am

Know thyself

As you do unto the least of these my brethren you do unto me

The pure in heart

But let a man examine himself, and so let him eat of that bread, and drink of that cup

Ye are gods

If the light within thee be darkness, how great is that darkness

I WORK. This observation is a most telling one. My strongest act as a human being is to acknowledge my personal functioning. It is much easier for me as child to live out a temper tantrum with violent threshing about than it is for me to pay kind attention to the mental material of which all of such violence is an unconscious (involuntary) expression. In other words, it is my thinking and my feeling and my perceiving, undisguised as doing, which constitute the distinct workings of the mind of my human being. It is much easier for me to perform, to do things, to act, than it is to see that such doing is an unconscious living of my own mental material. The function of doing, acting in the coarse sense, allows me to express my mind in a way which is diluted, or watered down, by partial unconsciousness. Once I am able to sustain my thought and feeling as acknowledged mental content, of which dramatic acting out would be the diluted form, I am then no longer under compulsion to express them in this unrecognized, falsely asserted, physical (non-mental) fashion. That is a great insight. When I work myself at my desk all day, as an executive, I am all fagged out at night, maybe more so than my brother living his factory by doing so-called manual labor. But when will my fellow man in mental motion with his muscles see that? It has been helpful to consider thinking and feeling as economic minute forms of action; it is also helpful to consider action as an economic minute form of conscious mental life.

I realize that I work myself always and that I am always working for me.

I PRAY. My prayer may be accurately defined as the study and practice of myself in the living of self-adoration. It is wise for me to be careful about what I pray for, since in praying, I am also the one prayed to. I am helpfully particular about my meaning for prayer. All of my living, itself, may be healthfully conceived as prayer. I offer as my scientific self-supplication, the following: May I grow ever to see more and more clearly the truth that all I can grow is me and that all of me is divine. May I enjoy the blessing of seeing clearly the disadvantages in a holier-than-thou or healthier-than-thou habit of mind. May I see clearly that loss and gain are absolutely evenly distributed throughout all of my humanity. May I see clearly that I must grow all of the chains and all of the wings my brother human being grows. May I live myself sanely, that is, self-consciously, and thus deliver myself from the hazards of my indulged carelessness. May I realize that I must make the effort to see all of my living as divinely just living. Therefore, may I consider myself comprehensively since I must do as I please. Since I am the surveyor and the surveyed, may I be aware of the truth that any one point of view cannot contradict another, that agreement is an illusion. May I renounce living to my disadvantage and, to that end, may I be prudently sensitive to my painful signs of self-hurt. May I live all of my necessity as my own. May I have the courage to measure my readiness for living, and thereby prevent my being overwhelmed in my attempt to live myself prematurely. May I spare myself the deception of believing that I ever can do anything wrong in my life. Whatever *is,* is adorable, and it is divine to be human: therefore may I ever maintain my divine look. So be it.

XVIII. I ORIGINATE
MY QUOTATIONS

The devil can cite Scripture for his purpose.

SHAKESPEARE

*　　*　　*

Numbers can have nothing by themselves. What prop-erties, what virtue, can ten flints, ten trees, ten ideas, possess merely because they are ten?—VOLTAIRE

To be able to count one and mean one fully—that is mathematical genius. To be able to write the word "I," and mean I fully—that is literary genius. I deem my great-est good to be my *awareness* of my self-possession. This specific appreciation, to the degree that I live it, enables me to realize that my life is worth living. Truly my esti-mate of the value of my life is the product of my recog-nition of the comprehensiveness of my individuality. In order to survive, I have had to hurt myself with my words ever since first learning to use words. Worst of all, I have alienated one part of my life which I designated "I" from every other part of my life which I would nominate "you,"

"he," "she," "it," "we," "they," or some other term implying not-I.

*   *   *

*The art to love your enemy consists in never losing
sight of* man *in him. Humanity has power over all that is
human: the most inhuman still remains man and never
can throw off all taste for what becomes a man—but you
must learn to wait.*—JOHANN KASPAR LAVATER

My only possible convincing means for seeing man in
my enemy or friend is seeing my selfness as constituting all
which I live as enemy or friend. My scientific method for
dealing with any and all of my psychic reality is founded
upon my clear realization that it *is* mine.

*   *   *

*The greatest truths, like the worst lies, the most sublime
discoveries and the most hideous errors of a people usually
grow from seeds that are not recognized for what they are;
they are brought to life by influences that are often looked
upon as the opposite of what they are. Therefore the physician who wants to cure evil should seek it in the ground;
but it is precisely when he seeks it there that the child or
the sick century turns against him. If he stoops to the level
of the cherished malady and seeks to cover it with a web
of health—who is greater and more welcome than he? He
is the pillar of all science and all fame. But the moment he
reaches out for our hearts, for our cherished ideas and
foibles which made us feel so comfortable—down with
him, the traitor to mankind, the murderer of our most
beloved truths and greatest joys!*—HERDER

It is not sufficient that I practice what I preach. Only

by practicing without preaching can I avoid the troubles of coercive education. The conceptions which develop the science of self-consciousness are the products of the renunciation of self-ignoration. Loving recognition of my every thought, word, deed, and omission, as being nothing but a creation of my own living, is an absolute requirement for my wholesome process of self-development. Being devoted to helping myself the best way I can, I naturally expect and wish (my) fellow man to help himself the best way *he* can.

* * *

The station we occupy among the nations of the earth is honorable, but awful. Trusted with the destinies of this solitary republic of the world, the only monument of human rights, and the sole repository of the sacred fire of freedom and self-government, from hence it is to be lighted up in other regions of the earth, if other regions of the earth ever become susceptible of its genial influence.

—THOMAS JEFFERSON

As an American patriot, instead of living my nationalism as a cult, I live my United States government as the best means for developing myself as a world citizen. I live my American citizenship; I live my world citizenship. Self-government recognizes the sovereignty of the individual. As a sovereign individual my responsibility is to learn how to reign well.

* * *

The chief disadvantage of knowing more and seeing farther than others is not to be generally understood. A man is, in consequence of this, liable to start paradoxes, which immediately transport him beyond the reach of the common-place reader. A person speaking once in a slighting manner of a very original-minded man received for answer—He strides on so far before you, that he dwindles in the distance.—WILLIAM HAZLITT

Emerson observed, to be great is to be misunderstood. True magnanimity includes the insight that all understanding is self-understanding. Only I can ever understand me. This comprehensive self-orientation makes possible the pacifying realization that any claim that one can understand or misunderstand another is pure illusion.

*   *   *

The great purpose of a college education is to enable a man to see cheerfully.—MILO H. GATES

All living is learning. All experience is self-experience. I do not have a number of life difficulties. My one life hardship is that of developing my capacity of self-tolerance. Of my life, that which I live cheerfully I live well.

*   *   *

For as that which is divine cannot be unfolded to the multitude, this mandate forbids the attempt to elucidate it to anyone but him who is fortunately able to perceive it.
—PLOTINUS

Here Plotinus is speaking of the perceiver and the perceived as being one, of his seeing or vision as being greater than, and prior to, his reasoning.

*   *   *

Attention, concentration, what you will, is one of the most remarkable mental functions. Not only can the meta-

phor of intense illumination of a particular field be justly used of it, but we may say that it seems to accelerate the flow of mental process through a particular channel, and so to draw into that channel the contents of other channels in connection with it, just as a rapid flow of water through a pipe sucks in water from connected pipes.

—JULIAN HUXLEY

My attention can be only my attention to my living of myself, can be only my self-consciousness. The health point is this: if I concentrate, study, attend, or use my mind's capacity for observation in any way, without realizing that such activity is my own mental activity, I thereby create mental disorder for myself.

*　　*　　*

The laws of science are, as we have seen, products of the creative imagination. They are the mental interpretations —the formulae under which we resume wide ranges of phenomena, the results of observation on the part of ourselves or of our fellow-men. The scientific interpretation of the phenomena, the scientific account of the universe, is therefore the only one which can permanently satisfy the aesthetic judgment, for it is the only one which can never be contradicted by our observation and experience. It is necessary to strongly emphasize this side of science, for we are frequently told that the growth of science is destroying the beauty and poetry of life.—KARL PEARSON

It is only the extension of my consciousness of myself which frees my imagination and provides me with a proper sense of its limitless possibilities.

*　　*　　*

As I have often emphasized, all great achievements of science start from intuitive knowledge, namely, in axioms, from which deductions are made.—ALBERT EINSTEIN

For my wholesome recognition of my life's worth, I must be able to realize that every element of my living is native to me, is a natural growth of my own. Everything which passes for my education is seen truly by me only when it is observable as my development *from within out.* Thus, I must grow the self-tolerance which enables me to appreciate that my environment is just as much a burgeoning of my life process as is my hand or my eye. Thus, I must develop the kind of self-endurance which arranges for me to claim that what my eye sees is as much my living as is my eye itself.

*   *   *

The way in which the mind creates new ideas is extremely complex. At the present time, notwithstanding important advances made in psychology, the study of mental activity has not yet enabled scientists to reach in their conclusions any agreement comparable to that reached in the older sciences. There is one aspect of the problem which should be of great interest to the student of our present civilization. The rapid growth in the technique and methods of scientific investigation and discovery has created a general belief that such discovery is made only by the systematic study of "cold facts" and by methodical reasoning. This belief is not entirely correct.

—C. W. THOMAS

The way in which the mind creates new ideas piques my curiosity in the same sense that I find myself profoundly interested in the nature of the way in which I grow any and every part of me. For the purpose of my establishing clearly my life's worth, all I need to know is that I am the creator of all of it. This self-consciousness is the solvent which is needed to dissolve my hard and cold facts so that I see them in my life's solution.

*   *   *

The same situation confronts the physicist everywhere; whenever he penetrates to the atomic or electronic level in his analysis, he finds things acting in a way for which he can assign no cause, for which he never can assign a cause, and for which the concept of cause has no meaning, if Heisenberg's principle is right. This means nothing more nor less than that the law of cause and effect must be given up.—P. W. BRIDGEMAN

The principle of individuality, clearly seen, requires the renunciation of the historic law of science designated as the law of determinism. Ascribing individuality to cause necessitates its being seen as its own effect; attributing individuality to effect necessitates its being seen as its own cause.

*   *   *

Science is probably unfavorable to the growth of litera- ture because it does not throw man back upon himself and concentrate him as the old belief did; it takes him away from himself, away from human relations and emotions, and leads him on and on. We wonder and marvel more, but we fear, dread, love, sympathize less. Unless, indeed, we finally come to see, as we probably shall, that after science has done its best the mystery is as great as ever, and the imagination and the emotions have just as free a field as before.—JOHN BURROUGHS

Thus my Burroughs speaks of the lack of the personal feelings in research work as delimiting the value of that effort. He designates such scientific dispassion, or apathy, as unhealthy. All of living is properly accessible for scientific growth. There can be no science which is not a scientist's living of it. For the scientist to live his passions composedly undoubtedly contributes to the distinctness of his sensory and perceptual living. How to live is as essential a question for my scientist as it is for my anyone. Conscious self-knowledge lengthens my life as a scientist; unconscious self-knowledge shortens my life as a scientist.

*　　*　　*

Nothing better shows the human self than the fact that we make an "I" of any material object which embodies, for the time being, our interest and purpose in the game of life; as a golf player will say, "I am in the creek beyond the hole." And if we call the body "I" it is only when we enter that too in the game, as when one says, "I am the tallest man here."—CHARLES HORTON COOLEY

To be able to identify myself in all of my conscious living is to be able to appreciate my life to the full.

*　　*　　*

> *Thought is deeper than all speech—*
> *Feeling deeper than all thought;*
> *Soul to soul can never teach*
> *What unto itself was taught.*
> —CHRISTOPHER P. CRANCH

Insofar as I recognize my education as entirely my self-activity I find it natural to renounce the illusions, I can tell somebody else something and somebody else can tell me something. In my ability to imagine my living as entirely my own lies my ability to imagine that my fellow man's living is all his own.

*   *   *

Between father and son there should be no reproving admonitions to what is good. Such reproofs lead to alienation, and than alienation there is nothing more unauspicious.—MENCIUS

Reproof implies the illusion: what is ought not be. My inability to recognize my every immaturity as the necessary stepping stone to my maturity is itself an immaturity which I need to live with love.

*   *   *

Good and evil do not wrongly befall men, because Heaven sends down misery or happiness according to conduct.—CONFUCIUS

I cannot drift, or coast, into mature health and strength. Only by disciplining myself in a way which necessitates it can I cultivate my human power.

*   *   *

No profit grows where is no pleasure ta'en:
In brief, Sir, study what you most affect.
—SHAKESPEARE

To the extent that I live my fellow man as troublesome, I ignore my true trouble which consists of my inability to recognize that my fellow man is living up to the extreme limits of his present ability.

*   *   *

In the awakening of consciousness life begins to be aware of its own limitless possibilities.—EDMOND HOLMES

I cannot exercise my self-consciousness without a sense of awe about the extent of my greatness.

*   *   *

The good critic is he who relates the adventures of his soul among masterpieces.—ANATOLE FRANCE

I am the critic and the criticized. My criticism enjoys all the benefits of humaneness, to the extent that I recognize it as nothing but comment upon phases of my own living.

*   *   *

The scientist is perhaps only a passing phase in the evolution of man; after unguessable years it is not impossible that his work will be done, and the problems of mankind will become for each individual the problem of best ordering his own life.—P. W. BRIDGEMAN

In losing my consciousness that my life is my own, my sense of being a person thereby disappears. Every sane moment of self-recognition serves me best for ordering my life.

*   *   *

Facts are popularly regarded as antidotes to mysteries. And yet, in sober earnest, there is nothing so mysterious as a fact.—L. P. JACKS

My scientific enlightenment occurred when I realized

the relief afforded by self-consciousness (self-insight) and the fact that I have the power of growth in self-consciousness. The mystery of my every fact is nothing but the mystery of my life which creates each fact.

* * *

Reality is that which explains itself and needs nothing else to explain it.—SPINOZA

Whatever is is all about itself and can have nothing to do with anything else (which is). Evidence can be nothing but self-evidence. I can bear witness to nothing but my own living.

* * *

As for ambition, what is it but a desire for an existence in the minds of other people—a desire which when fulfilled is a mockery, and unfulfilled a tomb?—EDGAR SALTUS

My safe and sane ambition is to grow myself consciously. This employment of my ambition saves me from attention seeking in that I find all of my attention where it really exists, in my consciousness of my self.

* * *

If democracy is flouted, what remains? There was a Greek proverb, "If water chokes, what can one drink to stop choking?" If the light of democracy be turned to darkness, how great is that darkness!—JAMES BRYCE

My political theory based upon my political ideal of self-government necessarily attributes sovereignty (self-government) of individuality to every human being of my world. However, the ideal of self-government is not a matter of preference, for whether or not I realize it I have no choice other than to live all of my own government. It is well to preface every allusion to self-government with the qualification "conscious." Thus: conscious self-government. The only possible political distinction which I can claim for myself is based upon whether or not I am conscious of my necessary self-government.

* * *

The primitive man is conservative in an extreme degree. Even on contrasting higher races with one another, and even on contrasting different classes in the same society, it is observable that the least developed are the most averse to change.—HERBERT SPENCER

The fact that my conscious cultivation of myself is left entirely up to me is a fact which merits my most careful caring and continuing appreciation. My developing myself so that I can skillfully and lovingly lift and operate myself is my vital issue which can concern only me. Whether or not I make myself consciously mindful is, and can be, only my concern. The more I attend insightfully to the world of me, the greater becomes my ability to mind my own business. Indispensable for my willingness to try to live the trials and tribulations of growing myself up self-tolerantly is the clear recognition that all of my tolerance is self-tolerance. The more I have experienced conscious self-tolerance and thereby its associated self-benefit, the more I see advantage in attempting further conscious self-tolerance.

XIX. MY MYTH OF HUMAN CRUELTY

*I know of no more encouraging fact than the unques-
tionable ability of man to elevate his life by conscious
endeavor.*

HENRY DAVID THOREAU

I OFTEN find expressed the idea that it is the nature of
man to be cruel and ferocious; that war must ever be, as
long as there are human beings; that "man's inhumanity
to man" is a necessity of his nature. All of this viewpoint
(advanced by such common sense beings as Hobbes and
Hume) depends for its validity on the principle that one
human being can have something to do with another human being. Man's fundamental nature is that of loving
kindness, indeed, that of adoration for all of his living.
What makes it possible for me to appear to be unkind, is
my lack of sensitiveness that it is myself that I am hurting
when I am having *my* fellow man hurt. If I extend my
self-consciousness to include more of my being, I, thereby,
proportionately increase my living kindly.

It is truly impossible for me to live myself other than
kindly in view of the fact that my individuality is naturally
concerned with all of my self-care. My living kindly may

be expressed in two ways: as evident kindness and as disguised kindness nominated "unkindness." My self-unkindness is the issue of my self-unconsciousness and the truest index of the degree to which I am unable to call my soul my own. This life-saving orientation is the creation only of self-insight. The conduct of my life, which includes the activity of the organs of my body in exactly the same sense that it includes the activity of the organs of my society, can be enlightened kind conduct only insofar as I am capable of feeling the truth that a help, or a harm, to any one of my organs (somatic or social) is lived as a help, or a harm, by every other one of my organs (somatic or social).

My every man tries his soul with his every day. My every man is basically friendly. My every man is naturally a man of peace. My every man depends upon his self-unconsciousness in his accounting for his psychology of war or for his hostility of any kind. My every man depends upon his self-consciousness in his accounting for his psychology of peace or for his humaneness of any kind. Only to the extent that I am a self-conscious individual can I devote my human energy to keeping the peace.

"Life can never be pleasant without virtue" was a fixed maxim of my Epicurus. My Coleridge pointed out, "Both in what we should do, and in what we should abstain from, the dictates of virtue are the very same with those of self-interest."

The "philosophy of sound common sense" (my John Locke), insofar as it asserts empiricism to be the origin of all knowing and all knowing to be an activity of the will, has a reality in it which only a comprehensive view of human individuality can provide. (My) every person's cruelty is indeed his effort to help himself by disposing of the hurt (he is feeling) in a part of himself where he cannot feel it (in *his* "other" part). My cruelty is nothing but my own imposed unkindness, necessitated by my own imposed unconsciousness that I am living myself painfully whenever I indulge my illusion that I can hurt another, or that my other one can hurt me. Quite as my Voltaire saw it, "Great crimes are always committed by great ignoramuses."

It is my due to live myself consciously, in the same sense that I deem it my due to breathe my air. Living my life according to a principle of self-ignoration is a suffocating kind of experience, but I escape feeling the cruelty of it once I succeed in forgetting it by willfully living it as not mine.

Sometimes it is most difficult for me to see the extent to which my self-love must be served by pain. Nevertheless I have found it desirable to make this truth a first principle of mine. Every sign or symptom of disease, disorder, abnormality, or pathology, is in truth a sign of health. Without such healthy signs denoting danger to my life, the possibility of recuperation would be eliminated.

XX. MY MORALITY DERIVES FROM MY SENSE OF SELF-BENEFIT

The pressure of autocratic authority tends to externalise life. The verdict of authority—external, visible, embodied authority—takes the place of the verdict of experience, of life, of nature. An officer's or a teacher's estimate of worth is accepted as final and decisive. An examiner's certificate determines a man's "station and degree." Class lists, orders of merit, prizes, medals, titles, grades, and the like interpose themselves between the soul and the ultimate realities of existence. Under such a régime the sense of intrinsic reality is gradually lost. What he is reputed to be is a man's chief concern, not what he really is. Now the intrinsically real has another name—the ideal.

EDMOND HOLMES

As a STUDENT of a certain way of developing myself, for instance, as a student of myself in my medical way of life, it behooves me to live every bit of my authorities, professors, patients, or what not, as nothing but my own living of it.

The cultivation of self-consciousness (recognized selfishness) is the cultivation of morality in its one and only workable sense: the advantage of *all of one,* and thus of one's all. However, as the matter of morality now stands it wobbles—the morality of mankind in general does not rest upon self-sight. Without awareness that I am injuring myself, I can apply thinly disguised self-punitive measures, all of the way from fines and imprisonment to capital punishment. I fine someone and claim it has nothing to do with myself. I execute someone and claim it is not any of my own life I am considering. Moral egoism and moral selfishness involve individual heroism. Such individual heroism is my only prescription for preventing such colossal stupidities of mine. Unkindness in any form is nothing but a defect of my self-consciousness. I can make the best of all of my unpleasantnesses only by seeing that the best is in each of them, the best in the form of notifying myself that I am hurting myself.

A heap of benefit comes to me when I can see what happens if I am loyal to this one doctrine of my individuality: to each his own everything, every man for his total self alone. There is nothing moral except what is of human benefit, and there is nothing human except all of my individuality. If I can be faithful to that! Of all the backslidings of my history, of all the falling away from my moral tenets, the one most costly to human life is: Do something for or against someone else. The doctrine of helping somebody else represents human sacrifice in my present day, for such depersonalization may be viewed as a form of human sacrifice. I observe this hangover of human sacrifice every hour. Thus self-exploitation, instead of self-devotion, is my fashionable education of my day.

The identity of self-sacrifice and self-exploitation is

hardly ever heeded. Shall I have altruism based upon my cruelty to myself, in the form of self-sacrifice—as though my other one were cruel enough to condone or even require (his) self-cruelty? Or shall I make peace with altruism based upon my own acknowledged self-devotion? Shall I assume healthy responsibility for self-devotion or sick guilt for my self-sacrifice? Which is preferable, the illusion of charity or the life of charity? The answer is such a self-evident truth that there must be some terrific opposition in the way to prevent my every one from seeing it at once. It is as if I would go to a mountain range and say, "Look at that mountain." And I would have my companion reply, "What mountain?," thus living a negative hallucination. How am I going to cherish this fundamental health doctrine of *taking care of all of myself* so that I will not succumb to the temptations to concern myself with an illuded something else or somebody else? My human physiology is doing harm to itself except to the extent that it senses development of itself. I aim to renounce talking about the physiology of somebody else at the expense of having my own physiology go to smash.

It is to my advantage to treat not only my everybody, but also my everything, well, that is, with love. Every man is his own, is his everything. Consciousness of his natural powers enables him to renounce demoralizing feelings of not amounting to much in his life course. Sensing his otherness as his own makes it the live issue which it is. It is as though what I can call "I," or "me," thereby becomes alive to me. The mental action through which mature love is demonstrated is conscious self-love. To devote my attention to anyone or to anything is to demonstrate my caring in terms of him or it by consciously living him or it as my own living. All I can really do when I say, "I attend to someone," is to live my meanings of someone as accurately as possible as my own. Thus the proposition, "Giving is getting," may be proved. So-called "giving of myself" always gets me greater selfness. "Love thy neighbor as thyself," rather than being a commandment, is an accurate observation. (My) everyone practices a modification of the golden rule. I do treat my others as I wish to treat myself. Trouble may lie in my inattention to my wish to hurt myself unprofitably. Thus I properly view running amuck as a form of treating the other fellow as I please. If I disown my need to hurt myself, that need can run wild, particularly in the realms of my self which I miscall "others."

Thomas Sydenham, my great physician who was much of a trial to his contemporaries, wrote, "T'is none of my business to inquire what other persons think, but to establish my own observations; in order to which, I ask no favor of the reader but to peruse my writings with temper." In Galatians VI, 4 and 5, I read, "Let every man prove his own works and then shall he have rejoicing in himself alone and not in another, for every man shall bear his own burden." "Those who trust us educate us," wisely noted my George Eliot.

The greatest contribution ever made to his so-called scientific knowledge is a man's profound and luminous enlightenment that all knowledge is self-knowledge. In my free United States of America my national doctrine of live and let live has deeper health significance than I may at first imagine it to possess. This health doctrine, now being lived by my reader, is all that I have been able to help myself with, and I intend to work upon it.

A teacher's work with *his* (self) student is essentially that of growing and integrating his own mental material. As far as his influence upon others is concerned, the mature educator has grown to renounce such an idea and sees it only as his own material. In my studying, I first exercise an individuation of myself (my lesson) and then see it as an integral part of the living of my all inclusive self.

In view of powerful and obvious motives to personal awareness of integration and self-interest, affecting all of the interests of my every individual, there can be nothing left but distrust of my mental maturity (or health or both) when I, in any quarter, oppose it. Most unfortunate of all is my violent endeavor to furnish make-believe ground for characterizing myself as a split personality, comprised of both selfness and otherness, and thus excite the illusion that there is a real difference of interests of two organized factions. Misrepresentation of the singleness of individuality is the only possible human mistake, but it occurs every which way. Nobody, nothing (no meaning of mine) can be alien to me. All of the people are inhabitants of each of the people. This singular figure of a human being, his mentally erect posture, is strongest of all. The only real ties that bind mankind exist *within* each man.

I have sense organs which inform me of myself only— what I am like, what pleasures and pains me, what helps and harms me, what is happening to me, what I grow to recognize as my appreciation of my everything (of me) I am experiencing. As individual, I note, I cannot have sense organs which inform me of anything but myself. Thus I observe that I am always living an environment which is also, necessarily, of my own making.

I work with the theory that it is impossible for me to consider fully, or point directly towards, my full pleasure before I can consider myself fully. To the extent that all of myself enters into the determination of what is pleasant, my pleasure principle may be seen to align with my reality principle. It is not sufficient that I am feeling good. I need to feel good about how I am living me, and that implies considering myself fully. As already observed, I cannot speak for all of myself at any given moment. The realization of that fundamental truth explains every apparent inconsistency, untruthfulness, infidelity, and all cognate changing of my mind. It also explains the need for my devoting myself steadily to the redeeming of my pledge or the keeping of my covenant.

I often deprive myself of my full measure of joy of life on account of my lack of appreciation of my wonderful ideas and feeling of anxiety, guilt, misery, despair, distrust, hatred, surrender, carelessness, weariness, and general inadequacy, of overwhelming myself with panics of such feelings. My St. John of the Cross comments sanely, "In all circumstances, however hard they may be, we should rejoice, rather than be cut down, that we may not lose the greatest good, the peace and tranquility of our soul. If the whole world and all that is in it were thrown into confusion, disquietude on that account would be a vanity, because that disquietude would do more harm than good." Awareness of distressing mental material like this (complete uselessness, hopelessness and general failure) is necessary to the development of awareness of thoroughly tested and true self-confidence, hope, love and happiness. For example, it is following awareness of mental material connoting self-loss, such as "I've gone as far as I can," "I give up," "What's the use," "You can't help me at all," "I'm worse than ever," "I don't care," that there occurs awareness of mental material connoting self-gain. Hence, by attending to most hopeless material hopefully, most anxious material courageously, and most hateful material lovingly, self-gain is felt.

Everyone grows his ability to control himself in his own unique way. As a rule, it appears that control is gained only by willfully esteeming inordinate fear of loss of control. Such an extreme dread of losing control is deadening to life itself, proscribing spontaneity and adventure essential for full living. Regaining my ability to lose control of myself, to the extent compliable with conscious fresh living, is a health necessity, if, for instance, I have identified loss of control only with loss of love.

It is perfectly evident to me, once I see distinctly, that every disadvantage I suffer is nothing but a helpful indicator to me that I have placed myself under living for which I am not yet fully ready, and a helpful director to me as to how to extricate myself. Everything is quite as it should be. It serves me right. All I can think about when I sense being in trouble is how to get out of it. Furthermore, without this sense, all my life would shortly disappear. I would not take long to end my life entirely if I were to deprive myself of my sense of disadvantage.

Whenever I act to my own ultimate disadvantage I am necessarily punishing myself, and any immediately sensed pleasure accruing from my short-sighted part-self indulgence is more apparent than is my unconsidered ultimate displeasure. However, as my awareness of my inclusiveness increases, I am forced to take more of myself under consideration habitually in the seeking of my pleasure. When I am aware that all has to do with me, it naturally follows: *my whole advantage* can offer pleasure to me when I am aware of my integration. My pleasure and reality principle merge economically towards my one goal: the attainment of life happiness in acting to my own best interests in increasing appreciation of myself.

The strategy of policing my morals must always defeat my purpose of promoting human dignity in that threats and promises, punishments and rewards, observed as coming from without, fan the flame of my human being's addiction to, preference for, externally imposed laws. My police force spares me the necessity to realize the work of *willing* my moral integration. Under the illusion of my external authority I can appear to myself to have my cake and eat it too. Thus I can force myself to appear to behave well without freely acknowledging any devotion to self-responsibility. My police force can dispense with evident consent and thus favor mental dissociation. Consciousness of the fact that I am *willing* all of my own living is indispensable to the growth of accurate and healthful awareness of my mental (including moral) integration.

Justice is not an experience reserved for a next world. Justice is a mortal value and a mortal experience. Every day is judgment day. I, here and now, have my day of reckoning. Nothing is more true of my psychic economy than that I pay as I go. I never owe anything. I never have credit. Each one of my (self) unkindnesses is costly, but I pay for it, fully. Each one of my investments is beneficial and pays dividends. I get what I pay for and only what I pay for. I get nothing for nothing. To accuse myself about any of my behavior is to indulge my pain-sparing illusion that I did not need to do what I did do, that I could just as well have done other than what I did.

I derive my only effective motivation for tempering my painful (unkind) emotion (such as hate, distrust, fear) when I fully understand that I can hurt myself with it. Only my anaesthetic hand is allowed to rest on my hot stove. I tend to renounce my lying when I add consciousness to the fact that I can only lie to myself. The same economic handling of my cheating, envying, lying, loving, and all the rest of my life sequences, follows my finding myself in this accurate way.

Only my mental faculties which can discern the distinction about degrees of self-help have full power of self-rule, of will. To attain full self-benefit requires full self-experience as to what is beneficial, and within my human being this experience is prescribed by vital functions such as sentience, percipience, and conscience (defined here as self-observation, as self-consciousness). I have created myself in such a way that I discriminatingly entrust my moral behavior to the propensions of my sensorium to select self-favoring experiences. The expression "common sense" carries some of this meaning. Nothing is competent to guide me, to carry my will, but that which naturally signifies my self-benefit. The moral import implicit in, and restricted to, the full definition of my human individuality is seldom observed, if I have not consistently trained myself in conscious self-interest.

Healthiest morality is not just a matter of appearing to do the right things. It includes my doing the right things in order to help myself most. It is a sign of my weak mind, immature or ill or both, that I must be offered more than this real basis for my socially acceptable behavior. The truest account for behaving myself well is that it is to my greatest advantage to care for myself. My wickedness consists of my degree of knowing no better than to hurt myself unprofitably, my degree of having to neglect my own gain. My very highest human ideal is the realization that all health is the issue of conscious self-development, the outcome of recognized self-growth.

If I observe that I am altogether, I can thereby find that my so-called contradictions, cross purposes, factions and partialities of all kinds are reconcilable selfness. Each of my particulars is all and only about itself. Any other view depends for acceptance upon distractibility. Not one of my meanings can be incompatible with my homogeneous selfhood. By virtue of the fact that I am a growing individual, therefore always a *one,* my selfhood never stops developing and thereby *discovering.* My seeing this truth is the road to accurate awareness of my mental integration.

The whole operation of the law of self-benefit depends upon the existence of self-consciousness. I can be most conscientious only when I am able to be conscious of most of myself. The quality of mercy is strained by the quantity of consciousness, for, after all, recognition of my need to be merciful with myself is channeled through my consciousness.

Seeing my experience as my own living of it is a necessary accompaniment of my good conscience. My whole mind can be conscientiously lived only to the extent that it is conscious. I can live my illusion of self-sacrifice with regard to any of my duties, obligations, offices, and so on, only by disregarding my truth that I am both recipient and sacrificer.

EPILOG: MY SONG OF MY
SELF-CONSCIOUSNESS

On the practical side of the question of egoism versus
self-surrender and for a trial of egoism in politics, this
may be said: the belief that men not moved by a sense
of duty will be unkind or unjust to others is but an in-
direct confession that those who hold that belief are
greatly interested in having others live for them rather
than for themselves. But I do not ask or expect so much.
I am content if others individually live for themselves and
thus cease in so many ways to act in opposition to my
living for myself.

J. L. WALKER

THERE FOLLOWS a series of observations, each of which is
chosen for its ability to highlight my introduction to living
consciously.

1. Consciousness of my personal identity, my I feeling, is
   my life's creation.
2. My awareness that I am exercises my appreciation of
   my life.
3. Observing that I am all me, my viewing my absolute

individuality insures the full coverage of my self-care.

4. I am growing myself. Living me is the extent of my human power. I am my own all, my own universe.

5. My individuality cannot be relational, all of my illusional between-ness is real within-ness; my every sensation, or perception, is entirely and only a self-development of mine.

6. I can live only my momentary surface selfness consciously; whole self can never be lived as a conscious experience.

7. I must live all of my life unconsciously except for my momentary surface consciousness of my selfness.

8. My orthodoxy is systematic devotion to my conscious self-development. All of my knowledge is self-knowledge, all of my ignorance is self-ignorance.

9. Only I can help myself, all help is self-help.

10. I cannot harm myself, all self-harm is unrecognized self-help.

11. My pain, evil, error, illness, injury, each is the helpful sign of manifest privation of its opposite, hence an indispensable aid to living myself well.

12. My vital mental powers, such as sensing, perceiving, conceiving, reasoning, and feeling, are products of my own creation which are lived consciously by me by means of my imagination.

13. Evaluating myself as divine is my highest self-estimate; evaluating myself as not divine is my lowest self-estimate.

14. I am gentle, kind, peaceful, and loving just so far as my self-consciousness can extend itself over my being.

15. Just so far as my self-consciousness restricts itself, I

tend to suffer neglect, or hurt, insensitively beyond the restricted zone.

16. To the extent that I can be a self-conscious person am I a peacemaker.

17. To the extent that I cannot be a self-conscious person am I a peacebreaker.

18. My extreme individualism constitutes my extreme sanity.

19. I can affirm only myself; I can negate only myself; my every word, or meaning, is a self-development of mine.

20. All of my world is alive, for I live it; all of my world is sensitive, for I live it.

21. Every experience of my life is most helpfully conceived by me as self-discovery.

22. My system of religion, philosophy, education, science, and psychology can be nothing but development of my human system.

23. My every meaning for "unlife" (inorganic, inanimate, non-vital, dead, non-viable) is in every respect *illusional*. All of my origin of all of my life is of my own origination. My problem of the origin of life is a phantom, traceable to my inability to realize and appreciate that all I can do is live. (My advent of my atomic age is helpful for my realizing and appreciating my atomic life. I have discontinued using the epithet "stone dead.")

24. My most helpful morality grows out of my most extended self-consciousness. Quite as my St. Augustine observed: Whatever is, is good.

25. I can test the depth of my sincerity by the amount of selfish interest I sense in it.

26. My feeling of being alone (all-one) is my most fundamental truth feeling.
27. My recognition of any problem of my world is essential for my seeing it as my own problem.
28. My ignorance, or ignoration, of any problem of my world cannot make it *no* problem of mine, cannot make it any less important for me.
29. I create myself; I create all of my own reality.
30. All of my language is essential for my self-definition and cannot be of any "other" use.
31. Creativity is natural; creativity is the only possible form of mental activity; conscious creativity is the only life there is in healthful pure science, or in any other revered originality, initiative, ingenuity, or recognized independent living of any kind.
32. Understanding is all and only self-understanding. I can neither understand nor misunderstand my very own creation which I designate "my fellow man." Either I must acknowledge that my fellow man's understanding must be all and only about himself, or I may vainly try to account for my inability to understand (my) him by such self-deceptions as "He is incomprehensible," "He is a mystic," even, "He is psychopathic."
33. *That I live* rather than *what I live* is the real basis for my life appreciation. To the extent that I can appreciate my life as such I can enjoy my mental health.

NAME INDEX

Name Index

SUBJECT INDEX

Subject Index

Subject Index

Mind, 1, 3
— change of, 2
— conflict, 53
— consciousness, 12, 30
— discipline, 11, 12, 50
— disorder, 25, 59
— dissociation, 12, 69, 86
— healing, 23, 78
— health, 1
— illness, 80
— immaturity, 80
— integration, 19, 70
— material, 89, 128, 131, 158
— modifications, 1
— object, 120
— strengthening, 23
— trauma, 77, 78, 123
— vs. matter, 58, 87
Misbehavior, 63
Morality, 130, 153–158, 167
Mother, 17, 18, 124, 125

Narcissism, 95
Necessity, 132
Negation, 83, 123, 124, 125
Neurology, 52
Not-I, 13, 14, 77, 105, 107, 109
Not-self, 52, 55, 68

Objectivity, 61
Orthodoxy, 22, 166
Otherness, 56

Pain, 16, 18, 22, 50, 51, 127, 128, 136, 149, 150, 151, 161, 166
Paradoxical cold, 47
Particular, 87
Past, 68
Pathology, 151
Peace, 6, 7, 27, 150, 167
Perception, 12, 24, 37, 38, 68, 71, 118, 119, 125, 166
Personal identity, 30
Phantasy, 12
Phantom, 49, 103, 132

Philautia, 95
Philosophy, 167
Physics, 58
Physiology, 38, 40, 50, 52, 54, 58, 106, 107
Pleasure principle, 158, 160
Plurality, 75, 137
Police force, 160
Practicality, 10, 62
Prayer, 135
Primitive humanity, 80
Psychic reality, 122
Psychoanalysis, 1
Psychology, 54, 58, 129

Reality, 16, 56, 117, 120, 147, 153
— principles of, 7, 158, 160
— testing, 24, 121, 122
Reasoning, 166
Religion, 91, 133, 167
Renunciation, 90, 107
Repression, 7, 22, 40, 52, 53, 86, 87, 96, 104
Research, 7, 8, 21
Resistance, 1, 5, 13
Responsibility, 17

Sanity, 26, 59, 62, 73, 88, 93, 128, 133, 158
Science, 2, 3, 10, 11, 12, 22, 29, 40, 117, 127, 141, 142, 144, 146, 167
— applied, 58
— definition of, 9
— experimental, 120
— method, 138
— of self, 3, 14, 23
— pseudo-science, 11, 12, 41
— scientific observation, 11
— scientific truth, 3
— scientist, 3
Scientific—method, 10
— imagination, 7, 113
Self, 12, 22
— activity, 1
— amnesia, 25, 28

173

Edited by Alexander Brede
Designed by Sylvia Winter
Set in Linotype Baskerville and Craw Clarendon
Printed on Warren's Olde Style Antique Wove
Bound in Bancroft's Linen Finished Cloth
Printed in the United States of America